The Quotable

OSLER

REVISED PAPERBACK EDITION

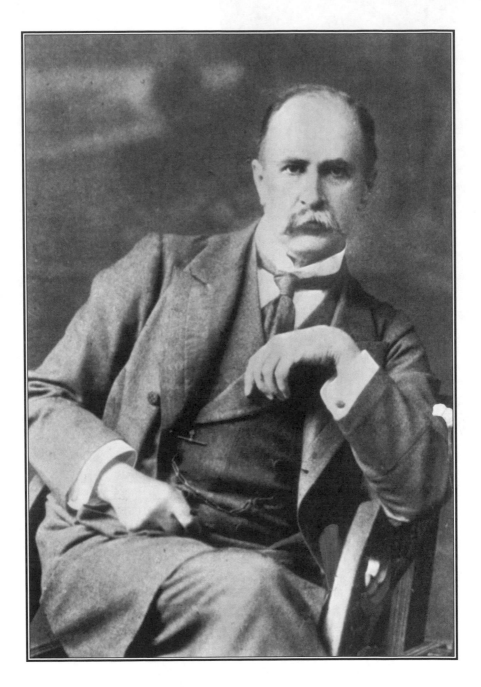

William Osler at Oxford in 1912.
(Courtesy of Earl Nation.)

The Quotable
OSLER

REVISED PAPERBACK EDITION

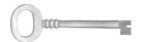

EDITED BY
MARK E. SILVERMAN, MD
T. JOCK MURRAY, MD
CHARLES S. BRYAN, MD

AMERICAN COLLEGE OF PHYSICIANS
PHILADELPHIA

Associate Publisher and Manger, Books Publishing: Tom Hartman
Production Supervisor: Allan S. Kleinberg
Senior Editor: Karen C. Nolan
Editorial Coordinator: Angela Gabella
Cover and Interior Design: Kate Nichols
Indexer: Kathy Patterson
Composition: Michael E. Ripca

Manufactured in the United States of America
Printing/binding by Versa Press

ISBN 978-1-934465-00-4

10 11 12 / 9 8 7 6 5

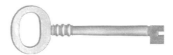

The latchkey represents the symbol of the American Osler Society. Osler gave latchkeys to several of his junior house staff (including Harvey Cushing) so they could have access to his home library in Baltimore. The favored house staff became known as the "latch-keyers."

Dedication

This revised edition of *The Quotable Osler*, like the first, is dedicated to John P. McGovern, MD, physician, scholar, and philanthropist. He was the principal founder of the American Osler Society, and his steadfast interest and substantial generosity over many years has greatly helped to keep the Oslerian spirit alive. After he read an advance copy, he wrote back: "Needless to say, your Preface is what struck me most, first were your 2 quotes, which are 2 of 3 that are my favorites, but my heart and head were inflamed on the second page wherein you and your co-authors so kindly dedicated this unique and splendid book to me. I truly can't put on paper the overriding love and joy that I felt. Swiftly my head said, Goodness, this book is a modern classic as soon as it comes off the press and surely will do much more to spread the Oslerian principles in the teaching and practice of medicine and life in general. Thank you from both head and heart for making me a part of it—I am grateful, plus."

Dr. McGovern died May 31, 2007.

Editors

Mark E. Silverman, MD, FACC, MACP, FRCP
Emeritus Professor of Medicine
Emory University School of Medicine
Chief of Cardiology, Fuqua Heart Center
Piedmont Hospital, Atlanta, Georgia

T. Jock Murray, OC, MD, FRCPC, MACP, FRCP
Professor Emeritus
Dalhousie University, Halifax, Nova Scotia

Charles S. Bryan, MD, MACP, FRCP(EDIN), FIDSA
Heyward Gibbes Distinguished Professor of Internal Medicine
Director, Center for Bioethics and Medical Humanities
University of South Carolina School of Medicine
Columbia, South Carolina

Contents

Foreword

Oslerian tags, quotes, and bon mots abound. Epigraphs by William Osler grace the pages of hundreds, probably many hundreds, of books and articles. So common is this form of flattery that people sometimes seem to find more in Osler than actually is there; frequently I am asked to identify "a bit of Osler," only to conclude after some investigation that another's pen must have written the questioned passage (though here as elsewhere it is awkward proving a negative).

Published collections of medical quotations make heavy use of Sir William. Maurice Strauss cites fifty-plus items in his anthology of 1968 (1) (Strauss in his *Index of Authors* does not itemize quotes for authors cited more than 50 times, of whom Osler is one), and the recent chrestomathy by Ed Huth and Jock Murray, *Medicine in Quotations* (2), finds space for 129.

Nevertheless, these numbers barely hint at the full menu of wisdom, common sense, and confection available in the voluminous writings of Osler. Thus this book.

Because this compilation directs its readers to cogent, and usually short, aphorisms rather than to lengthy quotations, an attempt to analyse Osler's writing style seems irrelevant here. For those interested in this approach to Osleriana there are a few references. One I wrote myself in 1969 as a rather cursory or preliminary treatment (3). More recently and definitively, Faith Wallis published "The Literary Styles of Sir William Osler" (4).

One predictable consequence flowing from the existence of this book is that the number of allusions to and quotations from Osler can only increase. Given that, the question that follows naturally has to be: is this A Good Thing? There are, after all, those few nay-sayers who find fault with a supposed adulation of William Osler, and who seem to think that he might now, eighty-plus years after his death, be ignored for more contemporary heroes. But the critics, aside from one or two instances of seriously flawed logic, seem to fall chiefly into the category of those who are uncomfortable beholding apparently seamless good sense, good humor, and good intentions, presented in good English.

And true enough, at times Osler can seem almost too good to be true. Yet surely cynicism should not rule here? It is telling, I believe, that Michael Bliss, Osler's current biographer, shared this feeling. He has recorded that when he began the research leading to his biography (5), he expected to find a darker side to the man. Yet when his work was finished, no darkness had been uncovered. As he put it: "Try as I might, I could not find a cause to justify the death of Osler's reputation" (6).

Many of us have favorite snippets of Osleriana to cherish and to reproduce at appropriate occasions. Three of mine are:

> "Though a little one, the masterword [Work] looms large in meaning. It is the open sesame to every portal, the great equalizer in the world, the true philosopher's stone which transmutes all the base metal of humanity into gold. The stupid man among you it will make bright, the bright man brilliant, and the brilliant student steady." (7)

And another, one that could apply to other professions as well, a sentence of eloquent succinctness coupled to sobering truth:

> "It is astonishing with how little reading a doctor can practise medicine, but it is not astonishing how badly he may do it." (8)

The solution, according to Osler, was simple:

> "With half an hour's reading in bed every night as a steady practice, the busiest man can get a fair education...." (9)

Such aphorisms convey assurance, confidence, and support to many who read or hear them. How could making such riches more readily accessible not be A Good Thing?

Charles G. Roland, MD
Heyward Gibbes Distinguished Professor of Internal Medicine
University of South Carolina School of Medicine

REFERENCES

1. Strauss MB, ed. Familiar Medical Quotations. Boston: Little, Brown; 1968.
2. Huth EJ, Murray TJ, eds. Medicine in Quotations: Views of Health and Disease Through the Ages, 2nd ed. Philadelphia: American College of Physicians; 2006.
3. Roland CG. Osler's writing style. JAMA. 1969;210:2257-60.
4. Wallis F. The literary styles of Sir William Osler. Osler Library Newsletter No. 51, February 1986.
5. Bliss M. William Osler: A Life in Medicine. Toronto: University of Toronto Press; 1999:xiv, 581.
6. Bliss M. William Osler: A Life in Medicine. Toronto: University of Toronto Press; 1999:xiii.
7. Osler W. The Master-Word in Medicine. In: Aequanimitas With Other Addresses to Medical Students, Nurses and Practitioners of Medicine. Philadelphia: P. Blakiston; 1928:373.
8. Osler W. Books and men. Boston Med Surg J. 1901;144:61.
9. Osler W. The medical library in post-graduate work. Brit Med J 1909;2:295-8.

Preface

*The practice of medicine is an art, not a trade; a calling, not
a business; a calling in which your heart will be exercised
equally with your head.*

*To study the phenomena of disease without books is to sail an
uncharted sea, while to study books without patients is not to
go to sea at all.*

*In taking up the study of disease, you leave the exact and cer-
tain for the inexact and doubtful and enter a realm in which
to a great extent the certainties are replaced by probabilities.*

SIR WILLIAM OSLER

Sir William Osler's teachings survive through his valued axioms that
capture the essence of the finest principles of medicine, education,
character, and philosophy of life. *The Quotable Osler* is an extensive selection of these sayings, published for the use of the many admirers of Sir
William who are seeking the apt quotation to enhance their articles or
lectures and for those readers who simply want to enjoy the inspiring
message of his humane and wise remarks. For those who may want to
know more about Osler, the man and his influence on medicine, we have
included an article by Richard Golden, written for the 150th anniversary
of Osler's birth, and have listed other useful sources below (1-11).

With the aid of the invaluable *Sir William Osler: An Annotated
Bibliography*, a listing of Osler's 1500 publications (7), and two previous
collections (8,9), the editors and members of the American Osler
Society have sifted through his writings for an observation or description
deemed to be original, wise, inspiring, educational, amusing, or of historical interest. Along the way, many little-known quotes of importance
were unearthed, and others, usually shortened into aphorisms, have
been restored to their full significance by being placed in context.

Since the first edition of *The Quotable Osler*, the Osler Library at
McGill University has discovered an unpublished, handwritten address
by William Osler, which he delivered to the University of Pennsylvania

entering class of 1885. From this manuscript, forty eloquent remarks have been added to this edition. This orientation address shows Osler, then only 36 years old, advising the young students how to develop the proper study habits that will carry them from the basic sciences through to their clinical responsibilities. At the same time, he emphasizes that "no two cases of the same disease are ever alike" and warns them "not to loose [*sic*] sight of the individual." Although some of these quotes may seem antiquated, they still retain a powerful message that the beginning student must learn to take care of the sick through an understanding of the basic sciences and the art of medicine.

The exhumation of this significant collection, ten more quotes from other sources, and the addition of a chronology of Osler's life justifies this softcover revised edition. We hope that it will be a gladly appreciated gift to a medical student, graduating resident, or even the veteran physician who stubbornly feels that Osler's teachings remain valuable today.

The quotations are sorted into nine major areas, each divided into sections. All quotations are numbered, and a short summary of each quote is provided. The extensive index refers the reader to the appropriate quotation number. Occasionally, bracketed comments are added within the quotations to clarify the source of Osler's literary references or to add needed explanation. Sir William's own literary influences were many and add a further dimension to his writing. References 10 and 11 provide an excellent resource for those interested in this subject. The source of each of quotation is given; frequently cited sources, such as *Aequanimitas*, have had their titles shortened in the text and complete bibliographical information moved to page 291. For all references without a stated author, Osler should be the assumed writer.

Because few women practiced medicine during Osler's period, some of his comments have a male gender orientation common to his time. These were understood then as an indefinite reference.

We are most appreciative of the enthusiastic help of the members of the American Osler Society listed below:

Charles T. Ambrose, Stanley E. Aronson, Steven L. Berk, Richard M. Caplan, Clifton R. Cleaveland, Barry N. Cooper, Burke A. Cunha, Martin L. Dalton, Paul G. Dyment, Lynn C. Epstein, Christopher G. Goetz, John T. Golden, Richard L. Golden, William S. Haubrich, Bruce J. Innes,

William H. Jarrett II, Richard J. Kahn, Robert C. Kimbrough III, Joseph W. Lella, Philip W. Leon, Neil McIntyre, William O. McMillan, Daniel E. Morgan, Earl F. Nation, Francis A. Neelon, Clyde Partin, Jr., Charles G. Roland, Clark T. Sawin, Barry D. Silverman, William A. Sodeman, Jr., Marvin J. Stone, Herbert M. Swick, Hector O. Venture, John B. West, Charles F. Wooley.

We gratefully acknowledge the invaluable organization skills and dedication of Linda Mason and Stacie Stepney, the careful editing of Diana Silverman and William Jarrett, and the Fuqua Heart Center at Piedmont Hospital. We especially acknowledge the late John P. McGovern, whose financial support contributed substantially to the launching of this project. Special thanks to Thomas Hartman and Karen Nolan, our excellent publishing editors for this edition; Joel Silverman and Tom Hyde for their photographic talent; and to the American College of Physicians…and, of course, our debt to Sir William Osler himself. May his spirit and lessons endure these troubling times.

Mark E. Silverman, MD
T. Jock Murray, MD
Charles S. Bryan, MD

REFERENCES

1. Golden RL. William Osler at 150: An Overview of a Life. JAMA 1999;282:2252-8.
2. Cushing H. The Life of Sir William Osler, 2 vols. Oxford: Clarendon Press; 1925.
3. Nation EF, Roland CG, McGovern JP. An Annotated Checklist of Osleriana, vols 1, 2. Montreal: McGill University of Osler Library; 2000.
4. Howard RP. The Chief: Doctor William Osler. Canton, MA: Science History Publications; 1983.
5. Bryan CS. Osler: Inspirations from a Great Physician. New York: Oxford University Press; 1997.
6. Bliss M. William Osler: A Life in Medicine. New York: Oxford University Press; 1999.
7. Golden RL, Roland CG. Sir William Osler: An Annotated Bibliography with Illustrations. San Francisco: Norman Publishing; 1988.
8. Camac CNB. Counsels and Ideals from the Writings of William Osler, 2nd ed. Boston: Houghton Mifflin; 1929.
9. Bean WB. Sir William Osler: Aphorisms from His Bedside Teachings and Writings, 3rd ed. Springfield, IL: Charles C Thomas; 1968.
10. Hinohara S, Niki H. Osler's "A Way of Life" and Other Addresses, with Commentary and Annotations. Durham, NC: Duke University Press; 2001.
11. Bryan CS. Saints of Humanity: Selections from Sir William Osler's Recommended Bedside Library. Columbia, SC: RL Bryan; 2002.

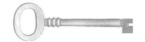

William Osler
at 150:
An Overview
of a Life

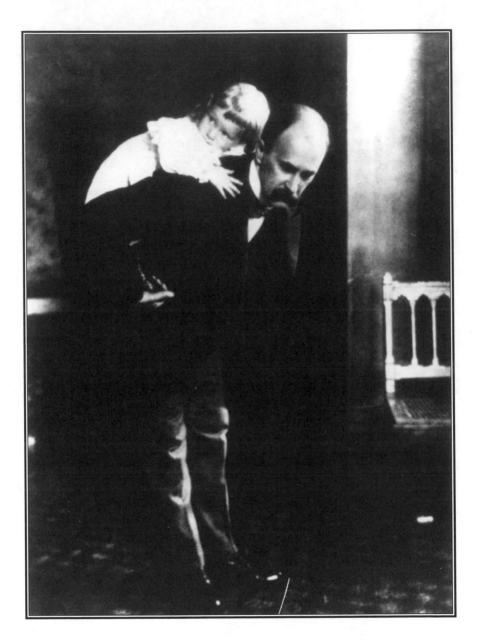

William Osler with 2-year-old son Revere, circa 1897.

RICHARD L. GOLDEN, MD

William Osler at 150: An Overview of a Life*

WILLIAM OSLER is among the most esteemed and distinguished physicians in the history of medicine.* His influence, clinical, educational, and literary, was global, and his legacy remains strong. He has been the subject of untold books, papers, essays, and tributes that continue unabated. Although Osler did creditable work in research, he was not a great scientist. The superlative may be applied to him as a clinician, but there were others who functioned at his level. Although tempting, it would be a semantic strain to call him a polymath. There are myriad notable achievers throughout history who are remembered only eponymically or as historical footnotes. Why, then, generations later, does the memory of Osler and his accomplishments continue to captivate succeeding generations?

Life

In reflecting on human achievement, the physician-writer (and Osler's favorite author) Sir Thomas Browne, observed: "But the iniquity of oblivion blindly scattereth her poppy and deals with the memory of men without distinction to merit of perpetuity. . . . Oblivion is not to be hired: The greater part [of men] must be content to be as though they

---

*Reprinted with modifications from JAMA 1999;282:2252-8. Used by permission of the American Medical Association. Copyright ©1999 by the American Medical Association.

had not been, to be found in the Register of God, not in the record of man" (1). Such was not to be Osler's fate, beginning with his birth at Bond Head, Ontario, on July 12, 1849, the anniversary of the Battle of the Boyne (1690) in which the forces of William III (Prince of Orange) defeated James II on the banks of the River Boyne, Ireland, in an important victory for the Protestant cause. When the celebrating Orangemen of this Irish Protestant district of Upper Canada marched to the parsonage in Bond Head, Osler's clergyman father appeared with the babe in his arms, and the crowd shouted "William" ("the little Prince of Orange"), and he was so christened.

As a youth, William showed considerable athletic and scholastic prowess, combined with high spirits and a reputation as a prankster. His escapades resulted in his expulsion from one school at the age of fourteen years and several days in jail two years later when he and his cronies barricaded the door of an unpopular school housekeeper and subjected her to the noxious fumes of molasses, pepper and mustard heated on the schoolroom stove (2)[p.22, 30-1].

Osler's initial undergraduate studies at Trinity College, Toronto were directed towards the ministry, following in the footsteps of his father. In Osler's second year, however, his keen interest in natural science, which had been strongly nurtured by his teachers, asserted itself in a decisive switch to medicine. He entered the Toronto Medical School and later transferred to McGill University School of Medicine, which offered a four-year curriculum and access to better clinical facilities at the Montreal General Hospital (2)[p71], (3)[p2]. After graduating in 1872, the newly minted doctor departed for the traditional European *wanderjahre* of Canadian graduates, with thoughts of a career in ophthalmology (2)[p91]. Osler pragmatically abandoned this quest when his friend and mentor, R. Palmer Howard, Professor of Medicine at McGill, wrote that other physicians in Montreal were planning to pursue this specialty. He then began to build the foundations for his future career with uncommonly broad-based studies that included physiology, medicine, pathology, surgery, neurology, and dermatology in the clinics and laboratories of London, Berlin, and Vienna.

Returning to his alma mater in 1874, Osler began an active period of teaching, private practice, performing autopsies, and taking charge of the dangerous smallpox wards for his willing colleagues. In addition to his formal lectures, he introduced the first course in clinical microscopy in Canada, purchasing the instruments at his own expense, and later established McGill's first physiology laboratory (2)[pp137,171], (3)[p4]. These unusually varied activities culminated in his appointment as professor of the Institutes of Medicine at McGill the following year. In 1878, he was elected to the post of attending physician at the Montreal General Hospital and at once began the practice of bedside teaching on his ward, a McGill tradition that contrasted with the predominantly didactic instruction at most medical schools of the time (4)[p59-60], (5,6).

In 1884, after tossing a coin to decide, Osler, with a firmly established and growing reputation, came to the United States as professor of clinical medicine at the University of Pennsylvania. He flourished in Philadelphia as teacher, clinician, and consultant, establishing a clinical laboratory at the University and imparting a contagious enthusiasm to students on the wards where he expanded bedside instruction and in the autopsy room where he demonstrated morbid anatomy (2)[pp235-6,252], (7). Osler also entered into the genteel social life of the city, participated in its clubs and societies, and established new friendships.

When John Shaw Billings offered Osler the chair of the department of medicine at the newly formed Johns Hopkins Hospital and Medical School in 1889, Osler did not hesitate to accept. This was the opportunity to fulfill his aspiration to establish a great clinic in the German model, with a well-organized house staff, proper laboratories and research, and an English system of clinical clerks (8,9). At Hopkins, a new era of American medicine was born, with rigorous admission requirements and a quality of training that set new standards in the United States and compared favorably with the venerable European institutions. Candidates for admission were required to have a four-year college degree, including two years of premedical training in biology, chemistry, and physics, and a reading knowledge of French and German (2)[p338]. The "Big Four" of Hopkins—William H. Welch in pathology and the future Dean, Osler in medicine, William S. Halsted in surgery, and Howard A. Kelly in gynecology—, all younger than 40 years, organized the hospital departments. Osler, in a jocular vein, commented to

Welch: "Well, we are lucky to get in as professors, for I am sure that neither you nor I could ever get in as students" (10).

It was at Hopkins that Osler wrote his *magnum opus* in 1891, *The Principles and Practice of Medicine* (11). The following year he married Grace Revere Gross, the widow of a Philadelphia friend and colleague, and a direct descendant of the Revolutionary War patriot Paul Revere. Legend has it that his unromantic proposal consisted of tossing the newly published book into her lap, saying: "There, take the darn thing, now what are you going to do with the man?" (2)[pp357-8].

Physically, Osler was of short stature by today's standards, lithe and brisk in movement, with a wiry athletic figure. Coal black hair over a high forehead, and penetrating dark brown eyes with a humorous twinkle, were engagingly set in a face of distinctive mobility that took on a serious, almost stern, aspect at rest. A large, black, flowing mustache and a peculiar, dark, almost olive complexion, reflective of his Celtic ancestry, added to his unique appearance. Dressed immaculately with a flower adorning the buttonhole of his dapper Prince Albert coat, he briskly arrived for rounds each morning leading his entourage with invariable good humor (12,13)[p118], (14,15).

In 1905, at the peak of his fame and under considerable stress from the burdens of teaching and practice, Osler was offered the Regius professorship of medicine at Oxford. Although the Chair at Oxford carried far fewer responsibilities, he hesitated in accepting this late career move. No doubt his positive decision was influenced by Mrs. Osler who cabled: "Do not procrastinate, accept at once. Better go in a steamer than go in a pine box" (16). With characteristic energy and verve, his tenure at Oxford, rather than being a sinecure, blossomed into a garland that capped an illustrious career. He organized clinics at the Radcliffe infirmary, founded journals and medical societies (17)[p49], and entered into the intellectual life of England with ultimate election to the presidencies of the Section of the History of Medicine of the Royal Society of Medicine (1912), the British Hospital Association (1913), the Fellowship of Medicine (1919), and the Ashmolean Natural History Society (1919).

His home at 13 Norham Gardens, with its continuous stream of visitors, became known as the Open Arms. Osler was created a baronet in

1911 as part of the coronation honors of George V. In 1917, his only surviving son, Revere, was tragically killed while serving in the British army, a blow that Osler struggled with for the remainder of his life. He wrote: "The Fates do not allow the good fortune that has followed me to go with me to the grave—call no man happy until he dies" (17)[pp577-8].

Sir William Osler died at Oxford in December 1919 of bronchopneumonia and empyema (18). In a biographical profile, the physician-historian Fielding H. Garrison said of him: "When he came to die, Osler was, in a very real sense, the greatest physician of our time. He was one of Nature's chosen. Good looks, distinction, blithe, benignant manners, a sun-bright personality, radiant with kind feeling and good will towards his fellow men, an Apollonian poise, swiftness and surety of thought and speech, every gift of the gods was his; and to these were added careful training, unsurpassed clinical ability, the widest knowledge of his subject, the deepest interest in everything human, and a serene hold on his fellows that was as a seal set upon them. His enthusiasm for his calling was boundless" (19).

He had served three nations, all of which took him for their own; a feat unlikely to bear repetition today.

Ethos

The distinguishing ethos of a man cannot be easily explained or divided into neat subdivisions, for there are nuances, interactions, and subtleties that defy precise analysis. Osler left a body of works encompassing writings in medical science and his philosophy of life, both personal and professional. In addition to his literary accomplishments, he was subject to the lure of bibliomania and built a magnificent library. He advanced the frontiers of medical education and was a unifying force in the medical profession. Osler had presence and a catalytic personality that brought him friendship, devotion, and disciples. But what was the binding force of this paradigm, the cement of the structure of his greatness? It was humanism. William Osler was a humanist, not merely in the narrow sense of educational or literary culture, which he certainly had, but in the broader sense of compassion, understanding, and the love of one's fellow man (20,21).

Writings

Osler left a vast written record, more than 1600 items encompassing medical, philosophical, educational and historical papers, essays, and books (22). As a young man of 19, fascinated with natural history and already a skilled microscopist, he published *Christmas and the Microscope* (23), a description of the microcosm of a winter stream near Dundas (Ontario) and the beginning of his "inkpot career" (24). While doing research in the London laboratory of Sir John Burdon-Sanderson, during his European post-graduate studies, Osler made important original observations on the nature of the blood platelet (25). On the wards, before the growth of specialization, his clinical perspicacity was legendary, and he was among the last of those giants who took all of medicine for their own.

Among the disorders that now bear or have borne his name are *Osler-Weber-Rendu disease* (hereditary hemorrhagic telangiectasia), *Osler disease* or *Osler-Vaquez disease* (polycythemia vera), *maladie d'Osler* or *Osler-Libman disease* (subacute bacterial endocarditis), and *Osler-Libman-Sacks syndrome* (systemic lupus erythematosus with verrucous endocarditis). Other terms with Osler's name include: *Osler maneuver* (pseudohypertension), *Osler phenomenon* (platelet agglutination), and *Osler nodes* (subacute bacterial endocarditis). Cushing suggested the nomenclature *Osler syndrome* for ball-valve gallstone with intermittent jaundice, chills, and fever. It is demonstrative of the catholicity of Osler's interests that there is also a trematode worm, found in the gills of a newt, that carries the name *Sphryanura osleri* and a nematode causing canine bronchitis, once called *Oslerus osleri* (13)[pp63-70].

Osler's single-authored textbook, *The Principles and Practice of Medicine*, went through 16 editions and influenced generations of students and practitioners for more than a half century, during which an estimated 500,000 copies were printed (26). Written in a clear, precise literary style with frequent classical and historical references, it provided the latest information on internal medicine enhanced by Osler's extensive knowledge of pathology. Unlike other textbooks, therapeutic information was limited and the absence of adequate treatment for most diseases freely admitted. The book's impact was not limited to the English-speaking world, which saw American, British, and Indian editions, but had a truly global effect through its translations into Russian, French, German, Chinese, Spanish, and Portuguese. In the summer of 1897, Frederick T. Gates, Baptist minister and philanthropic assistant to John D. Rockefeller, read the entire book to acquaint himself with the current state of medical knowledge. Impressed with the literary quality of the book and Osler's scientific candor on medicine's inability to cure most diseases, he recommended the support of medical research to Rockefeller. From this came the establishment of the Rockefeller Institute of Medical Research, a direct corollary of Osler's textbook (26).

Many a physician and scientist has left a distinguished and respected professional corpus but is little remembered by future generations. It was on the foundation of his nonscientific writings, however, that the conditions of Osler's special distinction began to take form. The best known of his philosophical essays, *A Way of Life* (27) and *Aequanimitas, With Other Addresses to Medical Students, Nurses and Practitioners of Medicine* (28), have been reprinted numerous times, the latter having been traditionally presented to some 150,000 graduating physicians between 1932 and 1953 (29). Here Osler tells us: "I have had three personal ideals. One to do the day's work well and not to bother about to-morrow. . . . The second ideal has been to act the Golden Rule, as far as in me lay, towards my professional brethren and towards the patients committed to my care. And the third has been to cultivate such a measure of equanimity as would enable me to bear success with humility, the affections of my friends without pride and to be ready when the day of sorrow and grief came to meet it with the courage befitting a man" (8).

With the *Titanic* in mind, he advises us to live with "day-tight compartments" (27)[pp11-6] and to follow the credo of Carlyle who said: "Your business is 'not to see what lies dimly at a distance, but to do what lies clearly at hand'" (30). He sets no lofty goals, suggests no pretentious achievements, but rather counsels us that, "To have striven, to have made an effort, to have been true to certain ideals—this alone is worth the struggle" (31).

Books and Libraries

With eloquence and wit, Osler acknowledged the extent of his bibliomania when addressing an international antiquarian booksellers congress: "You see before you a mental, moral, almost, I may say, a physical wreck—and all of your making. Until I became mixed up with you I was really a respectable, God-fearing, industrious, ardent, enthusiastic, energetic student. *Now* what am I? A mental wreck, devoted to nothing but your literature. Instead of attending to my duties and attending to my work, in come every day by the post, and by every post, all this seductive literature, with which you have, as you know perfectly well, gradually undermined the mental virility of many a better man than I" (32).

His lifelong devotion to books and libraries led to his election to the presidencies of the Medical Library Association [America] (1901), [England] (1910); the Bibliographical Society (1913); and the Classical Association (1919), uncommon achievements for a medical man. Osler's gifts to libraries were munificent and occasionally embarrassing, as when he absentmindedly presented a copy of Vesalius's *Fabrica* to McGill for the second time (17)[(p167)]. In the United States, his influence and untiring support were well known at the libraries of the Surgeon-General in Washington, the College of Physicians in Philadelphia, and at the Johns Hopkins Medical School and the Medical and Chirurgical Faculty in Baltimore. At Oxford, Osler served as ex-officio Curator of the Bodleian Library where he soon became a familiar face as both a dignitary and a reader (2)[(pp343-5)], (17)[(p43)]. When Osler spoke at the Boston Medical Library, he confessed: "It is hard for me to speak of the value of libraries in terms which would not seem exaggerated. Books have been my delight these thirty years, and from them I have received incalculable benefits" (33).

In the introduction to the *Bibliotheca Osleriana*, the descriptive catalogue of his great collection, Osler philosophizes: "a library represents the mind of its collector, his fancies and foibles, his strength and weaknesses and preferences. . . . The friendships of his life, the phases of his growth, the vagaries of his mind, all are represented" (24)[(ppxxi-xxxii)]. In the catalogue, Osler divides his library into eight divisions: "I. Prima, which gives in chronological order, a bio-biographical account of the evolution of science, including medicine; II. Secunda, the works of men who have made notable contributions, or whose works have some special interest, but scarcely up to the mark of those in Prima; III. Litteraria, the literary works written by medical men, and books dealing in a general way with doctors and the profession; IV. Historica, with the story of institutions, etc.; V. Biographica; VI. Bibliographica; VII. Incunabula; and VIII. Manuscripts" (24)[ppxxii-xxiii]. This collection of almost 8000 volumes was bequeathed to McGill University where it became the Osler Library of the History of Medicine in 1929.

The nucleus of the library is the Osler Niche, which is dominated by a bronze bas-relief of Osler, the Vernon Plaque, surrounded by his favorite books, including the works of Sir Thomas Browne, Robert Burton, and François Rabelais. Here, his ashes and those of Lady Osler lie concealed behind a panel in fulfillment of the bibliophilic desire of which he wrote: "I like to think of my few books in an alcove of a fire-proof library in some institution that I love; at the end of the alcove an open fire place and a few easy chairs, and over the mantle piece an urn with my ashes and my bust or my portrait through which my astral self, like the bishop of St. Praxed could peek at the books I have loved, and enjoy the delight in which kindred souls still in the flesh would handle them" (34,35)[pp91-114].

Education

In the field of education, Osler considered his advocacy of the bedside training of students as his major achievement and indeed suggested that his epitaph be "He taught medicine in the wards" (36). The dedication in Harvey Cushing's *The Life of Sir William Osler* is: "To Medical Students . . . lest it be forgotten who it was that made it possible for them to work at the bedside in the wards" (2)[pv]. At the Johns Hopkins Hospital, Osler introduced and utilized the clerkship as the means of clinical instruction and advocated that ". . . the natural method of teaching the student begins with the patient, continues with the patient, and ends his studies with the patient, using books and lectures as tools, as means to an end" (9).

In dealing with students, Osler not only correlated his teaching with ward work but opened his home and personal library and inculcated in them an interest in books and the history of medicine. Known as "the young man's friend" (37), he considered himself a life-long student and warned his pupils: "The hardest conviction to get into the mind of a beginner is that the education upon which he is engaged is not a college course, not a medical course, but a life course, for which the work of a few years under teachers is but a preparation" (38). To this end, Osler revealed to his students the "secret of life" promulgated in a single "master-word"—*work*. "To the youth it brings hope, to the middle-aged confidence, to the aged repose." He further elaborated: "The stupid man among you it will make bright, the bright man brilliant, and the brilliant student steady" (39).

Osler was well aware of the problems of medical education in his time and the major imperfections of many of the pre-Flexnerian medical schools where ill-prepared students received didactic instruction, often from poorly trained lecturers, in the context of an abbreviated curriculum (40)[(pp173-84)]. To this he counseled: "To study the phenomenon of disease without books is to sail an uncharted sea, while to study books without patients is not to go to sea at all" (33). In a day when students could graduate from medical school without having seen a delivery or the abdomen surgically opened, he urged his students to: "Live in the ward. Do not waste the hours of daylight in listening to that which you may read at night. But when you have seen, read. And when you can, read the original descriptions of the masters who, with crude methods of study, saw so clearly" (41).

Henry A. Christian, later professor of medicine at Harvard, recalled his student impressions of Osler at the bedside: "He would enter a ward . . . go to a patient's bed, . . . give him a cheery greeting and, if he were a new patient, ask for his history which was then given by the student clinical clerk. After it had been commented on, possibly criticized and often added to and illuminated by Dr. Osler . . . the report of the physical examination was called for from the clinical clerk. Often he was asked to demonstrate the features of the clinical examination. Usually Dr. Osler made some examination himself and demonstrated and discussed salient features, all the time mingling his discussion with remarks and explanations to the patient so that he would not be mystified or frightened. . . . Ward visits were an unusual combination of informality and dignity. Students and patients were quickly put at ease by Dr. Osler. His criticisms of students and their work were incisive and unforgettable, but never harsh or unkindly; they inspired respect and affection, never fear" (42).

Women were admitted to the new Johns Hopkins Medical School on the same basis as men as a result of the provisions of an endowment given by Mary Garrett, an ardent feminist (2)[pp373-4], (42)[p60]. Osler, who was sympathetic to the medical education of women, although with some reservations characteristic of the time, later wrote: "For years I have been waiting the advent of the modern Trotula [an 11th-century female medical author of Salerno], a woman in the profession with an intellect so commanding that she will rank with the Harveys, the Hunters, and Pasteurs; the Virchows, and the Listers. That she has not yet arisen is no reflection on the small band of women physicians who have joined our ranks in the last fifty years. Stars of the first magnitude are rare, but that such a one will arise among women physicians I have not the slightest doubt. And let us be thankful that when she comes she will not have to waste her precious energies in the worry of a struggle for recognition" (43,44).

Osler's approach to education was not only to produce technically competent physicians but extended to their personal lives in an effort to make reliable, caring physicians of high character and standards. He counseled medical students on "a way of life" (27), devised criteria and methods for their education (6), provided a textbook with both literary and scientific merit (11), and supported new schools and institutions. In a moving tribute, Wilder Penfield, the eminent Canadian neurosurgeon, said of him: "He belongs to medical students of all time, as Lincoln belongs to the common man everywhere, a man who grew to be what he wanted by dint of hard work, and in whose footsteps any undergraduate may dare to 'hope and dream' that he may follow" (45).

The Profession

Medicine was thought of in the divine sense by Osler when he poignantly told his students: "You are in this profession as a calling, not as a business; as a calling which exacts from you at every turn self-sacrifice, devotion, love and tenderness to your fellow-men. Once you get down to a purely business level, your influence is gone and the true light of your life is dimmed. You must work in the missionary spirit, with a breadth of charity that raises you far above the petty jealousies of life" (46). When he addressed the graduating class at McGill in 1875, he cited this lesson from his beloved hero, Sir Thomas Browne, cautioning that, "No one should approach the temple of science with the soul of a money changer" (47,48).

Osler was a peacemaker in the profession. He spread the doctrines of "unity, peace and concord" (49) among his colleagues by means of a personality that brooked no prejudice or intolerance, brought together clannish schools, societies and factions, and eliminated hostility through his special charm, friendship, and the appeal of a magnetic leadership. Just as early in his career he brought together the discordant French and English physicians of Montreal, so he later unified the medical community of Baltimore represented by five hostile medical schools that faced the perceived threat of the new Johns Hopkins Medical School (2)[p390]. On a national scale he called for a more cohesive profession by advocating interstate licensing reciprocity, medical school consolidation, and a reconciliation with homeopathists (in spite of "the anomaly of their position") (49).

In Oxford, bolstered by experiences in three nations, he helped draw together British and North American medicine. Osler strongly and repeatedly rejected contemporary medical chauvinism, proclaiming: "The great republic of medicine knows and has known no national boundaries" (39,50)[p111]. "The profession in truth is a sort of guild or brotherhood, any member of which can take up his calling in any part of the world and find brethren whose language and methods and whose aims and ways are identical with his own" (51).

Personality

An attempt to describe a personality is often an exercise in vacuous semantics, particularly in regard to the past. Osler lived in an early era of technology and probably left no vocal or cinematic clues, and, indeed, seemed ill at ease with the portraiture of canvas and camera. Nevertheless, it is from the narrations of his contemporaries and disciples, as well as his own words, that we garner some insights into this remarkable man. He had warm presence, a lodestone personality combined with charm and mirth, and the ability to effortlessly spread the mantle of his wisdom and friendship to a vast host. A New York pathologist, D. Bryson Delavan, sums up a more than 40-year acquaintanceship, describing Osler as: "Generous, gracious, magnetic, responsive, he attracted himself to all who were worth knowing, ever seeking merit in others and appreciating it when found. At once a discerning companion and a great leader, he more than others, has exemplified to me the beauty of friendship, the glory of work, and the joy of living" (52).

In reflecting on Osler's image, William B. Bean, first president of the American Osler Society, opined: "Though his warmth was widely diffused, it never became attenuated. Each person in the group—the patient, the nurse, the student—felt that Osler's special interest and favour centred on just one person, himself" (12).

Egerton Yorrick Davis was not only a *nom de plume* of Osler but a veritable alter ego who provided a balance and no doubt an outlet for the staid Victorian-Edwardian period in which he lived. It was in his Davis persona that Osler engaged in practical jokes, told tall tales, wrote elaborate hoaxes, and indulged his proclivities for sexual topics. He thus wrote on Peyronie's disease, penis captivus, and the fanciful marital and obstetrical customs of the Indian tribes of the Canadian Northwest Territories (35,53). Once, when in the throes of an attack of renal colic, he added some quartz stones from the driveway to his urine specimen (54). He often signed hotel registers as Egerton Y. Davis and playfully did so once while traveling with Mrs. Osler, no doubt to her annoyance and chagrin (2)[p578]. Henry Hurd, the first superintendent of the Johns Hopkins Hospital, observed: "His boyishness and love of fun continued as long as he remained in Baltimore, and many of his friends learned to know what to expect and to measure the amount of credence to be placed on many of his extravagant statements" (55).

A special facet of his personality was his delight in children who immediately sensed his empathy and affinity and allowed him uninhibited entry into their world. Wilder Penfield recalled his chilly reception as a student at Oxford University and his apprehensive arrival at the Open Arms to meet the Regius Professor: "At the far end of the room we found a young officer stretched out on the floor and Sir William on his knees bandaging an imaginary wound with his pocket handkerchief. The explanation of the strange scene was to be found in the ecstatic applause of two little children. They called the kneeling man William and he was evidently a beloved companion. He got up and came to me laughing" (56).

There are observers who consider that Osler's light-hearted, merry exterior concealed an inner melancholy and that his driving force flowed from a deep sorrow within, perhaps like "the wounded healer" of Aesculapian myth (11,13,57,58). Sir Robert Hutchinson believed that "a nature so sensitive as his could not escape from the sense of tears in mortal things and that his ears were always open to the 'sad still music of humanity'" (59). When asked why he whistled after attending a gravely ill patient, Osler replied, "I whistle that I may not weep" (60). The theory of his melancholy represents a minority view, provocative but uncorroborated.

Osler was remarkably free of prejudice, intolerance, and malevolence, particularly so, considering the contemporary mores to which he was exposed. In commenting on Osler's boyhood and the prejudices of the times, his cousin, Norman Gwynn, in a testament to a tolerance remarkable for the time, observed that "the seed of prejudice must have fallen on stony ground in Sir William's case. . . ." (61). This was echoed by Osler: "What I inveigh against is a cursed spirit of intolerance, conceived in distrust and bred in ignorance, that makes the mental attitude antagonistic, even bitterly antagonistic, to everything foreign, that subordinates everywhere the race to the nation, forgetting the higher claims of human brotherhood" (51). Commenting on the progress of the state of medicine in the English-speaking world, in a statement far ahead of his time, he further cautioned: "Distinctions of race, nationality, colour, and creed are unknown within the portals of the temple of Aesculapius" (62).

Sir Arthur S. MacNalty, who first met Osler as a student at Oxford, remembered him in this memorial tribute: "He advanced the science of medicine, he enriched literature and the humanities; yet individually he had a greater power. He became the friend of all he met—he knew the workings of the human heart metaphorically as well as physically. He joyed with the joys and wept with the sorrows of the humblest of those who were proud to be his pupils. He stooped to lift them up to the place of his royal friendship, and the magic touchstone of his generous personality helped many a disponder in the rugged paths of life. He achieved many honors and many dignities, but the proudest of all was his unwritten title, 'the Young Man's Friend'" (17)[pp685-6].

Humanism

Humanism is a complex, sometimes confusing, glibly used term; a catchword that may be loosely used to endorse the goals of various groups and individuals of diverse philosophies. It is used here not in its older and admittedly more precise educational and literary context, but in its more comprehensive sense. As Pellegrino has defined it: "Humanism encompasses a spirit of sincere concern for the centrality of human values in every aspect of professional activity. This concern focuses on the respect for freedom, dignity, worth, and belief systems of the individual person, and it implies a sensitive, non-humiliating, and empathetic way of helping with some problem or need" (63).

Humanism in the care of patients was not part of the contemporary idiom of Osler's era, but the concept was an innate part of his philosophy and professional conduct extending to his relationships with doctors, nurses, and students. He counseled the latter group to: "Care more particularly for the individual patient than for the special features of the disease" (50)[p97] . . . . "Nothing will sustain you more potently in your humdrum routine, as perhaps it may be thought, than the power to recognize the true poetry of life—the poetry of the common place, of the ordinary man, of the plain, toilworn woman, with their loves and their joys, their sorrows and their griefs" (38).

A cousin, Marian Osborne, Canadian author and poet, recounts how on a cold Montreal day Osler ran after an aged alcoholic beggar to whom he had earlier given some coins and, removing his overcoat, placed it on the astonished old man, exclaiming: "Here, take this, I have a father of my own. You may drink yourself to death, and undoubtedly will, but I cannot let you freeze to death" (60).

During his Oxford tenure, Osler was a frequent visitor to the home of his friend and colleague, Ernest Mallin. In a story oft-told, Dr. Patrick Mallam, then a child, recalls the illness of: ". . . a younger brother with very severe whooping-cough and bronchitis unable to eat and wholly irresponsive to the blandishments of parents and devoted nurses alike. Clinically it was not an abstruse case, but weapons were few, and recovery seemed unlikely" (64). Osler, on the way to graduation ceremonies in his academic robes, stopped and saw the child, and after a brief examination, peeled, cut, and sugared a peach, which he fed bit by bit to the enthralled patient. Although he felt that recovery was unlikely, he returned daily over a forty-day period, each time dressed in his doctors' robes, and personally fed the child some nourishment. Within a few days the tide began to turn and recovery became evident. Mallam concluded: "If the value of personal approach, the quick turning to effect of an accidental psychological advantage (in this case, decor), the consideration and extra trouble required to meet the needs of an individual patient, were ever well illustrated, here it was in fullest flower. It would, I submit, be impossible to find a fairer example of healing as an art. This kind of inspired magic, independent of higher degrees and laboratory gimmicks, is given only to a doctor with a real vocation, and the will to employ it" (64).

Summary

William Osler is the quintessential physician of our time because of his literary legacy, scientific and clinical accomplishments, educational contributions, and influence on intra-professional relations. He had an extraordinary personality, a facile wit, a bibliophilic spirit, and a philosophy of life that permitted him to envision and achieve remarkable goals. Osler's humanism, which permeated all of his activities, was the *sine qua non* of his particular claim to posterity. His continuing influence on succeeding generations is that of a role model (or hero in an older parlance) that has often been characterized as "the Oslerian tradition," a concept appropriately defined by Bryan as "a virtuous approach to medicine and life as taught and modeled by Osler" (65). The life and philosophy of William Osler continues to serve as a standard of excellence and a model for the evolution of the profession and its practitioners.

REFERENCES

1. Browne T. Hydriotaphia, or Urne Buriall. In: Endicott NJ, ed. The Prose of Sir Thomas Browne. Garden City, NY: Doubleday; 1967:282.
2. Cushing H. The Life of Sir William Osler. Oxford: Clarendon Press; 1925:i.
3. Howard RP. The Chief: Dr. William Osler. Canton, MA: Science History Publications; 1983.
4. Reid EG. The Great Physician: A Short Life of Sir William Osler. New York: Oxford University Press; 1931.
5. Howard RP. William Osler: "A Potent Ferment" at McGill. Arch Int Med 1949;84:12-5.

6. Osler W. License to Practice. Maryland Med J 1889;21:61-7.
7. Leidy J II. Student Reminiscences: Philadelphia Period. Int Assoc Med Mus Bull (Special Osler Memorial Number) 1926;9:218-21.
8. Osler W. L'envoi. In: Aequanimitas, With Other Addresses to Medical Students, Nurses and Practitioners of Medicine. Philadelphia: P Blakiston; 1906:469-74.
9. Osler W. The Hospital as a College. In: Aequanimitas, With Other Addresses to Medical Students, Nurses and Practitioners of Medicine. Philadelphia: P Blakiston; 1906:327-42.
10. Welch WH. Twenty-Fifth Anniversary of the Johns Hopkins Hospital, 1889-1914. Johns Hopkins Hosp Bull 1914;25:363-6.
11. Osler W. The Principles and Practice of Medicine. New York: D Appleton; 1892.
12. Bean WB. Osler: The Legend, the Man and the Influence. CMAJ 1966;95:1031-7.
13. Bett WR. Osler: The Man and the Legend. London: William Heinemann; 1951.
14. Thayer WS. Osler. Int Assoc Med Mus Bull (Special Osler Memorial Number) 1926;9:286-93.
15. Finney JTM. A Personal Appreciation of Sir William Osler. Int Assoc Med Mus Bull (Special Osler Memorial Number) 1926;9:273-85.
16. Bensley EH, Bates DG. Sir William Osler's Autobiographical Notes. Bull Hist Med 1976;50:596-618.
17. Cushing H. The Life of Sir William Osler. Oxford: Clarendon Press; 1925:ii.
18. Barondess JA. A case of Empyema: Notes on the Last Illness of Sir William Osler. Trans Am Clin Climatol Assoc 1975;86:59-72.
19. Garrison FH. An Introduction to the History of Medicine. Philadelphia: WB Saunders; 1929:631.
20. Knight JA. William Osler's Call to Medicine. John P. McGovern Award Lecture, Institute for the Medical Humanities, University of Texas Medical Branch. Galveston, 18 May 1983.
21. Roland CG. The Palpable Osler: A Study in Survival. Perspectives Biol Med 1984;27:299-313.
22. Golden RL, Roland CG. Sir William Osler. An Annotated Bibliography with Illustrations. San Francisco: Norman Publishing; 1988.
23. Osler W. Christmas and the Microscope. Hardwicke's Science-Gossip: An Illustrated Medium of Interchange and Gossip for Students and Lovers of Nature 1869;5:44.
24. Osler W. Bibliotheca Osleriana. Oxford: Clarendon Press; 1929.
25. Osler W. An Account of Certain Organisms Occurring in the Liquor Sanguinis. Proc Roy Soc 1873-74;22:391-8.
26. Golden RL. Osler's Legacy: The Centennial of *The Principles and Practice of Medicine*. Ann Int Med 1992;116:255-60.
27. Osler W. A Way of Life. New York: Oxford University Press; 1926.
28. Osler W. Aequanimitas, With Other Addresses to Medical Students, Nurses and Practitioners of Medicine. Philadelphia: P Blakiston; 1904.
29. Kimbrough RC III. The Good Gift: A Comparison of the Eli Lilly Presentation Copies of *Aequanimitas*. J South Carolina Med Assoc 1995;91:350-4.
30. Osler W. The Army Surgeon. In: Aequanimitas, With Other Addresses to Medical Students, Nurses and Practitioners of Medicine. Philadelphia: P Blakiston; 1906:103-20.
31. Osler W. An Alabama Student. In: An Alabama Student and Other Biographical Essays. London: Oxford University Press; 1908:1-18.
32. Osler W. Address Before the International Association of Antiquarian Booksellers at the Criterion Restaurant, Piccadilly, Jan. 26, 1911. Bookseller [London]; 1911:144-5.

33. Osler W. Books and Men. In: Aequanimitas, With Other Addresses to Medical Students, Nurses and Practitioners of Medicine. Philadelphia: P Blakiston; 1904:217-25.
34. Francis WW. At Osler's Shrine. Bull Med Lib Assoc 1937;26:1-8.
35. Davis EY. Burrowings of a Book-Worm. In: Golden RL, ed. The Works of Egerton Yorrick Davis, MD: Sir William Osler's Alter Ego. Osler Library Studies in the History of Medicine, No. 3; Montreal: McGill University; 1999:93-115.
36. Garrison FH. Osler's Place in the History of Medicine. Int Assoc Med Mus Bull (Special Osler Memorial Number) 1926;9:29-33.
37. Malloch A. Finch and Baines. Cambridge: Cambridge University Press; 1917:vii-viii.
38. Osler W. The Student Life. In: Aequanimitas, With Other Addresses to Medical Students, Nurses and Practitioners of Medicine. Philadelphia: P Blakiston; 1906:413-43.
39. W. The Master-Word in Medicine. In: Aequanimitas, With Other Addresses to Medical Students, Nurses and Practitioners of Medicine. Philadelphia: P Blakiston; 1904:363-88.
40. Ludmerer KM. Learning to Heal: The Development of American Medical Education. New York: Basic Books; 1985:173-84.
41. Thayer WS. Osler the Teacher. In: Osler and Other Papers. Baltimore: The Johns Hopkins University Press; 1931:1-5.
42. Christian HA. Recollections of an Undergraduate Medical Student at Johns Hopkins. Arch Int Med 1949;84:77-83.
43. Osler W. The Growth of a Profession. Can Med Surg J 1885-6;14:129-55.
44. Osler W. Dr Mary Putnam Jacobi. In: In Memoriam of Dr. Mary Putnam Jacobi. New York: Academy of Medicine; 1907:3-8.
45. Penfield W. Hero Worship. Arch Int Med 1949;84:104-9.
46. Osler W. The Reserves of Life. St. Mary's Hosp Gaz 1907;13:95-8.
47. Strauss MB. Familiar Medical Quotations. Boston: Little, Brown; 1968:406.
48. Osler W. Valedictory Address to the Graduates in Medicine and Surgery, McGill University. Can Med Surg J 1874-1875;31:433-42.
49. Osler W. Unity, Peace and Concord. In: Aequanimitas, With Other Addresses to Medical Students, Nurses and Practitioners of Medicine. Philadelphia: P Blakiston; 1906:445-65.
50. Bean RB, Bean WB. Sir William Osler: Aphorisms from His Bedside Teachings and Writings. Springfield, IL: Charles C Thomas; 1961.
51. Osler W. Chauvinism in Medicine. In: Aequanimitas, With Other Addresses to Medical Students, Nurses and Practitioners of Medicine. Philadelphia: P Blakiston; 1906:277-306.
52. Delavan DB. A Reminiscence of Sir William Osler. Int Assoc Med Mus Bull (Special Osler Memorial Number) 1926;9:202-4.
53. Nation EF. William Osler on Penis Captivus and Other Urological Topics. Urology 1973;2:468-70.
54. Futcher TB. Dr. Osler's Renal Stones. Arch Int Med 1949;84:40.
55. Hurd HM. The Personality of William Osler in Baltimore. Int Assoc Med Mus Bull (Special Osler Memorial Number) 1926;9:262-5.
56. Penfield W. A Medical Student's Memories of the Regius Professor. Int Assoc Med Mus Bull (Special Osler Memorial Number) 1926;9:385-7.
57. Singer C. Osler: Some Personal Recollections. Brit Med J 1949;2:46-7.
58. Dewey N. Sir William Osler and Robert Burton's *Anatomy of Melancholy.* JAMA 1969;210:2245-50.

59. Hutchinson R. William Osler. Quart J Med 1949;18:275-7.
60. Osborne M. Recollections of Sir William Osler. Int Assoc Med Mus Bull (Special Osler Memorial Number) 1926;9:171-4.
61. Gwyn NB. The Boyhood of Sir William Osler. Can Med Assoc J (Special Osler Memorial Number) 1920;10:24-7.
62. Osler W. British Medicine in Greater Britain. In: Aequanimitas, With Other Addresses to Medical Students, Nurses and Practitioners of Medicine. Philadelphia: P Blakiston; 1904:167-96.
63. Pellegrino ED. Humanism and the Physician. Knoxville: University of Tennessee Press; 1979:118.
64. Mallam P, Billy O. JAMA 1969; 210:2236-9.
65. Bryan CS. What is the Oslerian Tradition? Ann Int Med 1994;120:682-7.

I

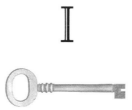

Personal Qualities

- ✢ Ideals and Character

- ✢ Equanimity and Detachment

- ✢ Philosophy, Goals, Blessings

- ✢ Charitableness, Speech, The Press

- ✢ Time Management and Work Ethic

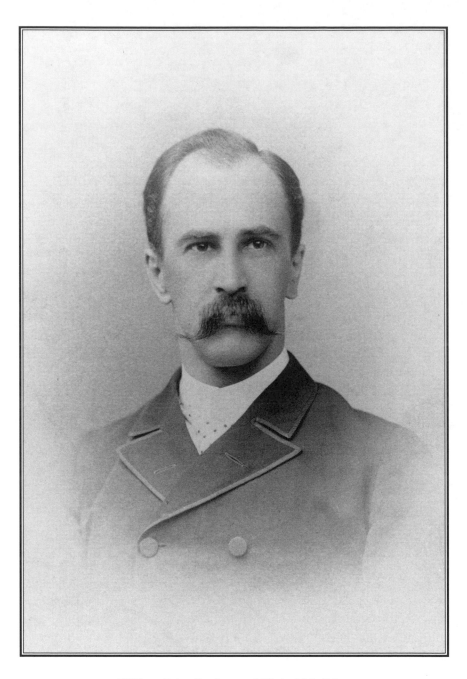

William Osler, Professor of Clinical Medicine,
University of Pennsylvania, circa 1887.
(Courtesy of the Osler Library of the History of Medicine,
Montreal, Quebec, Canada.)

Personal Qualities

Ideals and Character

1. Osler's personal ideals.

I have had three personal ideals. One to do the day's work well and not to bother about to-morrow. It has been urged that this is not a satisfactory ideal. It is; and there is not one which the student can carry with him into practice with greater effect. To it, more than to anything else, I owe whatever success I have had—to this power of settling down to the day's work and trying to do it well to the best of one's ability, and letting the future take care of itself. The second ideal has been to act the Golden Rule, as far as in me lay, towards my professional brethren and towards the patients committed to my care. And the third has been to cultivate such a measure of equanimity as would enable me to bear success with humility, the affection of my friends without pride and to be ready when the day of sorrow and grief came to meet it with the courage befitting a man.

L'ENVOI, IN AEQUANIMITAS, 450 1.

2. Have realizable ideals.

Not that we all live up to the highest ideals, far from it—we are only men. But we have ideals, which mean much, and they are realizable, which means more.

TEACHING AND THINKING, IN AEQUANIMITAS, 119.

3. Apply the Hippocratic standards—learning, sagacity, humanity, and probity.

To you the silent workers of the ranks, in villages and country districts, in the slums of our large cities, in the mining camps and factory towns, in the homes of the rich, and in the hovels of the poor, to you is given the harder task of illustrating with your lives the Hippocratic standards of Learning, of Sagacity, of Humanity, and of Probity. Of learning, that you may apply in your practice the best that is known in our art, and that with the increase in your knowledge there may be an increase in that priceless endowment of sagacity, so that to all, everywhere, skilled succour may come in the hour of need. Of a humanity, that will show in your daily life tenderness and consideration to the weak, infinite pity to the suffering, and broad charity to all. Of a probity, that will make you under all circumstances true to yourselves, true to your high calling, and true to your fellow man.

THE MASTER-WORD IN MEDICINE, IN AEQUANIMITAS, 370-1.

4. To be true to certain ideals is worth the effort.

To have striven, to have made an effort, to have been true to certain ideals—this alone is worth the struggle.

AN ALABAMA STUDENT, IN AN ALABAMA STUDENT, 18.

5. Old ideals still inspire.

The times have changed, conditions of practice have altered and are altering rapidly, but when such a celebration takes us back to your origin in simpler days and ways, we find that the ideals which inspired them are ours to-day—ideals which are ever old, yet always fresh and new, and we can truly say in Kipling's words:

> The men bulk big on the old trail, our own trail, the out trail,
> They're God's own guides on the Long Trail, the trail that is
>   always new.
>   [from "The Long Trail" by Rudyard Kipling (1865-1936)]
> On the Educational Value of the Medical Society, in Aequanimitas, 345.

6. Strive for the impossible.

Nothing in life is more glaring than the contrast between possibilities and actualities, between the ideal and the real. By the ordinary mortal, idealists are regarded as vague dreamers, striving after the impossible; but in the history of the world how often have they gradually moulded to their will conditions the most adverse and hopeless! They alone furnish the *Geist* [spirit] that finally animates the entire body and makes possible reforms and even revolutions. Imponderable, impalpable, more often part of the moral than of the intellectual equipment, are the subtle qualities so hard to define, yet so potent in everyday life, by which these fervent souls keep alive in us the reality of the ideal.

> Unity, Peace and Concord, in Aequanimitas, 428-9.

7. Choose between your own interest and ideals.

My message is chiefly to you, Students of Medicine, since with the ideals entertained now your future is indissolubly bound. The choice lies open, the paths are plain before you. Always seek your own interests, make of a high and sacred calling a sordid business, regard your fellow creatures as so many tools of trade, and, if your heart's desire is for riches, they may be yours; but you will have bartered away the birthright of a noble heritage, traduced the physician's well-deserved title of the Friend of Man, and falsified the best traditions of an ancient and honourable Guild. On the other hand, I have tried to indicate some of the ideals which you may reasonably cherish…. And though this course does not necessarily bring position or renown, consistently followed it will at any rate give to your youth an exhilarating zeal and a cheerfulness which will enable you to surmount all obstacles—to your maturity a serene judgment of men and things, and that broad charity without which all else is nought—to your old age that greatest of blessings, peace of mind, a realization, maybe, of the prayer of Socrates for the beauty in the inward soul and for unity of the outer and the inner man.

TEACHER AND STUDENT, IN AEQUANIMITAS, 40-1.

8. Protect your ideals.

And, if the fight is for principle and justice, even when failure seems certain, where many have failed before, cling to your ideal, and, like Childe Roland [from "Childe Roland to the Dark Tower Came" by Robert Browning (1812-1889)] before the dark tower, set the slug-horn to your lips, blow the challenge, and calmly await the conflict.

AEQUANIMITAS, IN AEQUANIMITAS, 8.

9. There are three lessons to learn.

Mastery of self, conscientious devotion to duty, deep human interest in human beings—these best of all lessons you must learn now or never.

SIR THOMAS BROWNE, IN AN ALABAMA STUDENT, 277.

10. Perfection is to be cultivated.

The artistic sense of perfection in work is another much-to-be-desired quality to be cultivated. No matter how trifling the matter on hand, do it with a feeling that it demands the best that is in you, and when done look it over with a critical eye, not sparing a strict judgment of yourself.

THE MASTER-WORD IN MEDICINE, IN AEQUANIMITAS, 362.

11. Judge exceptional men by different standards.

Exceptional men cannot be judged by ordinary standards.

THE TREATMENT OF DISEASE. CAN LANCET 1909;42:899-912.

12. The most dangerous foe is apathy.

By far the most dangerous foe we have to fight is apathy—indifference from whatever cause, not from a lack of knowledge, but from carelessness, from absorption in other pursuits, from a contempt bred of self-satisfaction.

UNITY, PEACE AND CONCORD, IN AEQUANIMITAS, 436.

13. Intellectual laziness is a vice.

The killing vice of the young doctor is intellectual laziness.

ON THE EDUCATIONAL VALUE OF THE MEDICAL SOCIETY, IN AEQUANIMITAS, 334.

14. Avoid complacency.

Maintain an incessant watchfulness lest complacency beget indifference, or lest local interests should be permitted to narrow the influence of a trust which exists for the good of the whole country.

BEAN WB. SIR WILLIAM OSLER: APHORISMS, 72.

15. *Pretending to know is a conceit.*

That greatest of ignorance—the ignorance which is the conceit that a man knows what he does not know.

CHAUVINISM IN MEDICINE, IN AEQUANIMITAS, 285.

16. *Self-satisfaction is comparable to a delusion of grandeur.*

Self-satisfaction, a frame of mind widely diffused, is manifest often in greatest intensity where it should be least encouraged, and in individuals and communities is sometimes so active on such slender grounds that the condition is comparable to the delusions of grandeur in the insane.

THE ARMY SURGEON, IN AEQUANIMITAS, 101-2.

17. *Ignorance increases dogmatism.*

The greater the ignorance the greater the dogmatism.

CHAUVINISM IN MEDICINE, IN AEQUANIMITAS, 284.

18. *Humility deserves a place of honor.*

In these days of aggressive self-assertion, when the stress of competition is so keen and the desire to make the most of oneself so universal, it may seem a little old-fashioned to preach the necessity of this virtue, but I insist for its own sake, and for the sake of what it brings, that a due humility should take the place of honour on the list.

TEACHER AND STUDENT, IN AEQUANIMITAS, 38.

19. *A sceptical attitude is an advantage.*

One special advantage of the skeptical attitude of mind is that a man is never vexed to find that after all he has been in the wrong.

THE TREATMENT OF DISEASE. CAN LANCET 1909;42:899-912.

20. *Common sense is rare before forty.*

Common-sense nerve fibers are seldom medullated before forty—they are never seen even with a microscope before twenty.

BEAN WB. SIR WILLIAM OSLER: APHORISMS, 134.

21. *We are at the mercy of our wills.*

We are at the mercy of our wills much more than our intellect in the formation of beliefs, which we adopt in a lazy, haphazard way without taking much trouble to enquire into their foundation.

THE TREATMENT OF DISEASE. CAN LANCET 1909;42:899-912.

22. *Physicians should be wary of professional arrogance.*

Perhaps no sin so easily besets us as a sense of self-satisfied superiority to others. It cannot always be called pride, that master sin, but more often it is an attitude of mind which either leads to bigotry and prejudice or to such a vaunting conceit in the truth of one's own beliefs and positions, that there is no room for tolerance of ways and thoughts which are not as ours are.

CHAUVINISM IN MEDICINE, IN AEQUANIMITAS, 270.

23. *Do not be too sensitive.*

We all belong to one or other of two groups, the *leiodermic*, with nice, soft, woolly skins, on which the pinpricks of life, though felt, make no serious impression: and the *algedermic*, with raw, painful skins, which every rough contact irritates. Unfortunately, it is very much a matter of temperament or inheritance, but from the start it makes a great difference if you are not too sensitive, not too ready to react to the irritations of life.

THE RESERVES OF LIFE. ST. MARY'S HOSP GAZ 1907;13:95-8.

24. Character influences character.

This higher education so much needed to-day is not given in the school, is not to be bought in the market place, but it has to be wrought out in each one of us for himself; it is the silent influence of character on character and in no way more potently than in the contemplation of the lives of the great and good of the past, in no way more than in "the touch divine of noble natures gone."

BEAN WB. SIR WILLIAM OSLER: APHORISMS, 83.

25. Books influence character.

Carefully studied, from such books come subtle influences which give stability to character and help to give a man a sane outlook on the complex problems of life.

SIR THOMAS BROWNE, IN AN ALABAMA STUDENT, 276-7.

26. Culture is helpful to physicians.

A physician may possess the science of Harvey and the art of Sydenham, and yet there may be lacking in him those finer qualities of heart and head which count for so much in life.... Medicine is seen at its best in men whose faculties have had the highest and most harmonious culture.

BRITISH MEDICINE IN GREATER BRITAIN, IN AEQUANIMITAS, 168-9.

27. Maintain a good humor.

Hilarity and good humour, a breezy cheerfulness, a nature "sloping toward the southern side," as Lowell has it [referring to the sunny side, from "An Epistle to George William Curtis" by James Russell Lowell (1819-1891)], help enormously both in the study and in the practice of medicine. To many of a sombre and sour disposition it is hard to maintain good spirits amid the trials and tribulations of the day, and yet it is an unpardonable mistake to go about among patients with a long face.

THE STUDENT LIFE, IN AEQUANIMITAS, 405.

28. Laughter brightens life.

Like song that sweetens toil, laughter brightens the road of life, and to be born with a sense of the comic is a precious heritage.

TWO FRENCHMEN ON LAUGHTER, IN MEN AND BOOKS, 9.

29. Laughter is the music of life.

Bubbling spontaneously from the artless heart of child or man, without egoism and full of feeling, laughter is the music of life.

TWO FRENCHMEN ON LAUGHTER, IN MEN AND BOOKS, 12.

30. Face disaster erect and with a smile.

Stand up bravely, even against the worst.... Even with disaster ahead and ruin imminent, it is better to face them with a smile, and with the head erect, than to crouch at their approach.

AEQUANIMITAS, IN AEQUANIMITAS, 8.

31. The yoke of conformity is inevitable.

Sooner or later—insensibly, unconsciously—the iron yoke of conformity is upon our necks; and in our minds, as in our bodies, the force of habit becomes irresistible. From our teachers and associates, from our reading, from the social atmosphere about us, we catch the beliefs of the day, and they become ingrained—part of our nature. For most of us this happens in the haphazard process we call education, and it goes on just as long as we retain any mental receptivity.

HARVEY AND HIS DISCOVERY, IN AN ALABAMA STUDENT, 299-300.

32. *The race of life requires capability and endurance.*

For final success the race winner must have reserves, not merely the capability and energy for the short run (such as that in which you have been engaged) but endurance or, as the expression is, staying powers.

THE RESERVES OF LIFE. ST. MARY'S HOSP GAZ 1907;13:95-8.

33. *To reach distinction from the top requires grit and a hard climb.*

Quite as much grit and a much harder climb are needed to reach distinction from the top as from the bottom of the social scale.

WILLIAM PEPPER, IN AN ALABAMA STUDENT, 212.

Equanimity and Detachment

34. *Cultivate a measure of obtuseness.*

Cultivate, then…such a judicious measure of obtuseness as will enable you to meet the exigencies of practice with firmness and courage, without, at the same time, hardening "the human heart by which we live." [from *Ode (Intimations of Immortality from Recollections of Early Childhood)* by William Wordsworth (1770-1850)]

AEQUANIMITAS, IN AEQUANIMITAS, 5.

35. *Don't complain unnecessarily.*

You may learn to consume your own smoke. The atmosphere is darkened by the murmurings and whimperings of men and women over the non-essentials, the trifles that are inevitably incident to the hurly burly of the day's routine. Things cannot always go your way. Learn to accept in silence the minor aggravations, cultivate the gift of taciturnity and consume your own smoke with an extra draught of hard work, so that those about you may not be annoyed with the dust and soot of your complaints.

THE MASTER-WORD IN MEDICINE, IN AEQUANIMITAS, 368.

36. Cultivate a cheerful heart.

The greatest gift that nature or grace can bestow on a man is the *aequus animus,* the even-balanced soul; but unfortunately nature rather than grace, disposition rather than education, determines its existence. I cannot agree...that it is not to be acquired. On the contrary, I maintain that much may be done to cultivate a cheerful heart.

ROBERT BURTON, IN A WAY OF LIFE, 87.

37. Knowing what to do provides imperturbability.

In a true and perfect form, imperturbability is indissolubly associated with wide experience and an intimate knowledge of the varied aspects of disease. With such advantages he is so equipped that no eventuality can disturb the mental equilibrium of the physician; the possibilities arc always manifest, and the course of action is clear. From its very nature this precious quality is liable to be misinterpreted, and the general accusation of hardness, so often brought against the profession, has here its foundation. Now a certain measure of insensibility is not only an advantage, but a positive necessity in the exercise of a calm judgment, and in carrying out delicate operations.

AEQUANIMITAS, IN AEQUANIMITAS, 5.

38. Sensitivity should not interfere with performance.

Keen sensibility is doubtless a virtue of high order, when it does not interfere with steadiness of hand or coolness of nerve; but for the practitioner in his working-day world, a callousness which thinks only of the good to be effected, and goes ahead regardless of smaller considerations, is the preferable quality.

AEQUANIMITAS, IN AEQUANIMITAS, 5.

39. Have your nerves in hand.

The first essential is to have your nerves well in hand. Even under the most serious circumstances, the physician or surgeon who allows "his outward action to demonstrate the native act and figure of his heart in complement extern," [from *Othello* by William Shakespeare (1564–1616)] who shows in his face the slightest alteration, expressive of anxiety or fear, has not his medullary centres under the highest control, and is liable to disaster at any moment.

AEQUANIMITAS, IN AEQUANIMITAS, 4.

40. Imperturbability is an important quality.

In the first place, in the physician or surgeon no quality takes rank with imperturbability.... Imperturbability means coolness and presence of mind under all circumstances, calmness amid storm, clearness of judgment in moments of grave peril, immobility, impassiveness, or, to use an old and expressive word, *phlegm*. It is the quality which is most appreciated by the laity though often misunderstood by them; and the physician who has the misfortune to be without it, who betrays indecision and worry, and who shows that he is flustered and flurried in ordinary emergencies, loses rapidly the confidence of his patients.

AEQUANIMITAS, IN AEQUANIMITAS, 3-4.

41. Equanimity is difficult to obtain but necessary.

Let me recall to your minds an incident related of that best of men and wisest of rulers, Antoninus Pius [2nd century Roman emperor], who, as he lay dying, in his home at Lorium in Etruria, summed up the philosophy of life in the watchword, *Aequanimitas*. As for him, about to pass *flammantia moenia mundi* [the flaming ramparts of the world], so for you, fresh from Clotho's spindle [a Greek goddess, youngest of the three Fates, who spun the thread of human life], a calm equanimity is the desirable attitude. How difficult to attain, yet how necessary, in success as in failure!

AEQUANIMITAS, IN AEQUANIMITAS, 5-6.

42. Equanimity enables you to overcome the trials of life.

It has been said that "in patience ye shall win your souls," and what is this patience but an equanimity which enables you to rise superior to the trials of life? Sowing as you shall do beside all waters, I can but wish that you may repeat the promised blessing of quietness and assurance forever, until

> Within this life,
> Though lifted o'er its strife...
> [from "Rabbi Ben Ezra" by Robert Browning (1812-1889)]

you may, in the growing winters, glean a little of that wisdom which is pure, peaceable, gentle, full of mercy and good fruits, without partiality and without hypocrisy.

AEQUANIMITAS, IN AEQUANIMITAS, 8.

43. Do not expect too much from others.

One of the first essentials in securing a good-natured equanimity is not to expect too much of the people amongst whom you dwell.... Deal gently then with this deliciously credulous old human nature in which we work, and restrain your indignation.

AEQUANIMITAS, IN AEQUANIMITAS, 6.

44. Equanimity is bearing with composure the distress of others.

It has been said that in prosperity our equanimity is chiefly exercised in enabling us to bear with composure the misfortunes of our neighbours.

AEQUANIMITAS, IN AEQUANIMITAS, 7.

45. Humility gives permanence to powers.

The Art of Detachment, the Virtue of Method, and the Quality of Thoroughness may make you students, in the true sense of the word, successful practitioners, or even great investigators; but your characters may still lack that which can alone give permanence to powers—*the Grace of Humility.*

TEACHER AND STUDENT, IN AEQUANIMITAS, 37.

46. Acquire the art of detachment.

In the first place, acquire early the *Art of Detachment,* by which I mean the faculty of isolating yourselves from the pursuits and pleasures incident to youth. By nature man is the incarnation of idleness, which quality alone, amid the ruined remnants of Edenic characters, remains in all its primitive intensity. Occasionally we do find an individual who takes to toil as others to pleasure, but the majority of us have to wrestle hard with the original Adam, and find it no easy matter to scorn delights and live laborious days.

TEACHER AND STUDENT, IN AEQUANIMITAS, 33.

47. The art of detachment is a precious gift.

A rare and precious gift is the Art of Detachment, by which a man may so separate himself from a life-long environment as to take a panoramic view of the conditions under which he has lived and moved: it frees him from Plato's den long enough to see the realities as they are, the shadows as they appear. Could a physician attain to such an art he would find in the state of his profession a theme calling as well for the exercise of the highest faculties of description and imagination as for the deepest philosophic insight.

CHAUVINISM IN MEDICINE, IN AEQUANIMITAS, 265.

48. Stay calm.

Educate your nerve centres so that not the slightest dilator or contractor influence shall pass to the vessels of your face under any professional trial.

AEQUANIMITAS, IN AEQUANIMITAS, 4.

Philosophy, Goals, Blessings

49. We are influenced by those we admire.

Not by the lips, but by the life, are men influenced in their beliefs.

SCIENCE AND IMMORTALITY, 37.

50. Love humanity through love of your profession.

The love of humanity associated with the love of his craft! – philanthropia and philotechnia – the joy of working joined in each one to a true love of his brother.

THE OLD HUMANITIES AND THE NEW SCIENCE. BOSTON:HOUGHTON MIFFLIN
Co.;1920:63.

51. *The wisdom of tomorrow is the foolishness of yesterday.*

The philosophies of one age have become the absurdities of the next, and the foolishness of yesterday has become the wisdom of to-morrow.

CHAUVINISM IN MEDICINE, IN AEQUANIMITAS, 266.

52. *The philosophy of practical life is to know what to do.*

To know just what has to be done, then to do it, comprises the whole philosophy of practical life.

BRITISH MEDICINE IN GREATER BRITAIN, IN AEQUANIMITAS, 171.

53. *Pursue a cherished purpose by tenacity of will.*

To few is given the tenacity of will which enables a man to pursue a cherished purpose through a quarter of a century...to fewer still is the fruition granted.

BOOKS AND MEN, IN AEQUANIMITAS, 209.

54. *Life's race is hard and short with help at hand.*

In ordinary training you run the course over, but life's race is run but once; and, though, the course may seem long to you, it is really very short, but very hard to learn. Fortunately, you are not alone on the track, as your brothers are ahead, and if you are willing there is always help at hand.

THE RESERVES OF LIFE. ST. MARY'S HOSP GAZ 1907;13:95-8.

55. *View life from two points.*

From two points of view alone have we a wide and satisfactory view of life—one, as, amid the glorious tints of the early morn, ere the dew of youth has been brushed off, we stand at the foot of the hill, eager for the journey; the other, wider, perhaps less satisfactory, as we gaze from the summit, at the lengthening shadows cast by the setting sun. From no point in the ascent have we the same broad outlook, for the steep and broken pathway affords few halting places with an unobscured view.

AFTER TWENTY-FIVE YEARS, IN AEQUANIMITAS, 191.

56. Life is a habit.

A few years ago a Xmas card went the rounds, with the legend 'Life is just one "derned" thing after another,' which, in more refined language, is the same as saying "Life is a habit," a succession of actions that become more or less automatic.

A WAY OF LIFE, IN A WAY OF LIFE, 238.

57. Three lessons are to be learned from Thomas Browne.

There are three lessons to be gathered from the life of Sir Thomas Browne [(1605-1682), physician who attempted to reconcile scientific skepticism and faith in his 1643 book *Religio Medici*], all of them of value to-day. First, we see in him a man who had an ideal education.... The second important lesson we may gain is that he represents a remarkable example in the medical profession of a man who mingled the waters of science with the oil of faith.... The third lesson to be drawn is that the perfect life may be led in a very simple, quiet way.

CUSHING H. THE LIFE OF SIR WILLIAM OSLER, VOL. 2, 24-5.

58. Plan ahead.

When schemes are laid in advance, it is surprising how often the circumstances fit in with them.

INTERNAL MEDICINE AS A VOCATION, IN AEQUANIMITAS, 138.

59. *A calm life is necessary for continuous work.*

The truth that lowliness is young ambition's ladder is hard to grasp, and when accepted harder to maintain. It is so difficult to be still amidst bustle, to be quiet amidst noise; yet...the calm life [is] necessary to continuous work for a high purpose.

TEACHER AND STUDENT, IN AEQUANIMITAS, 39.

60. *There are two types of great leaders.*

There are two great types of leaders; one, the great reformer, the dreamer of dreams—with aspirations completely in the van of his generation—lives often in wrath and disputations, passes through fiery ordeals, is misunderstood, and too often despised and rejected by his generation. The other, a very different type, is the leader who sees ahead of his generation, but who has the sense to walk and work in it. While not such a potent element in progress, he lives a happier life, and is more likely to see the fulfillment of his plans.

WILLIAM PEPPER, IN AN ALABAMA STUDENT, 211.

61. *Be in charge and be glad you are alive.*

Prepare to lay your own firm hand upon the helm. Get into touch with the finite, and grasp in full enjoyment that sense of capacity in a machine working smoothly. Join the whole creation of animate things in a deep, heartfelt joy that you are alive, that you see the sun, that you are in this glorious earth which Nature has made so beautiful, and which is yours to conquer and to enjoy.

A WAY OF LIFE, IN A WAY OF LIFE, 243.

62. *Appreciate your blessings and advantages.*

It is a common experience that men do not always appreciate their blessings and advantages. Those who are the best off are the least sensible of it.

THE GROWTH OF A PROFESSION. CAN MED SURG J 1885-1886;14:129-55.

63. *Find happiness through work and colleagues.*

Happiness comes to many of us and in many ways, but I can truly say that to few men has happiness come in so many forms as it has come to me. Why I know not, but this I do know, that I have not deserved more than others, and yet, a very rich abundance of it has been vouchsafed to me.... I have had exceptional happiness in the profession of my choice, and I owe all of this to you. I have sought success in life, and if, as some one has said, this consists in getting what you want and being satisfied with it, I have found what I sought in the estimation, in the fellowship, and friendship of the members of my profession.

L'ENVOI, IN AEQUANIMITAS, 447.

64. *Friends, colleagues, and pupils promote success.*

To have had the benediction of friendship follow me like a shadow, to have always had the sense of comradeship in work without the petty pinpricks of jealousies and controversies, to be able to rehearse in the sessions of sweet, silent thought the experiences of long years without a single bitter memory fill the heart with gratitude. That three transplantations have been borne successfully I owe to the brotherly care with which you have tended me. Loving our profession and believing ardently in its future I have been content to live in it and for it. A moving ambition to become a good teacher and a sound clinician was fostered by opportunities of exceptional character and any success I may have attained must be attributed in large part to the unceasing kindness of colleagues and to a long series of devoted pupils whose success in life is my special pride.

DAVISON WC. SIR WILLIAM OSLER: SIR WILLIAM OSLER: REMINISCENCES. ARCH INT MED 1949;84:110-28.

Charitableness, Speech, The Press

65. Have patience and charity towards others.

Curious, odd compounds are these fellow-creatures, at whose mercy you will be; full of fads and eccentricities, of whims and fancies; but the more closely we study their little foibles of one sort and another in the inner life which we see, the more surely is the conviction borne in upon us of the likeness of their weaknesses to our own. The similarity would be intolerable, if a happy egotism did not often render us forgetful of it. Hence the need of an infinite patience and of an ever-tender charity toward these fellow-creatures; have they not to exercise the same toward us?

AEQUANIMITAS, IN AEQUANIMITAS, 6.

66. Be aware of your own frailties.

Dealing as we do with poor, suffering humanity, we see the man unmasked, or so to speak, we see him in his uniform, exposed to all the frailties and weaknesses, and you have got to keep your heart pretty soft and pretty tender not to get too great a contempt for your fellow creatures.

ADDRESS TO THE STUDENTS OF THE ALBANY MEDICAL COLLEGE. ALBANY MED ANN 1899;20:307-9.

67. Say nothing if not complimentary.

If you cannot say anything good about a man, say nothing.

PRATT J. OSLER AS HIS STUDENTS KNEW HIM. BOSTON MED SURG J 1920;182:338-41.

68. Success depends on attitude.

Not only will your success in life, but your happiness depend upon the attitude of mind which you habitually assume towards your fellow-creatures.

THE RESERVES OF LIFE. ST. MARY'S HOSP GAZ 1907;13:95-8.

69. Don't overestimate yourself.

Enjoying the privilege of wide acquaintance with men of very varied capabilities and training, you can, as spectators of their many crochets and of their little weaknesses, avoid placing an undue estimate on your own individual powers and position.

THE ARMY SURGEON, IN AEQUANIMITAS, 102.

70. Don't act superior.

Shun as most pernicious that frame of mind, too often, I fear, seen in physicians, which assumes an air of superiority, and limits as worthy of your communion only those with satisfactory collegiate or sartorial credentials. The passports of your fellowship should be honesty of purpose, and a devotion to the highest interests of our profession, and these you will find widely diffused, sometimes apparent only when you get beneath the crust of a rough exterior.

THE ARMY SURGEON. MED NEWS [PHILADELPHIA] 1894:318-22.

71. *Your own frailties make you considerate of others.*

Keep a looking glass in your own heart, and the more carefully you scan your own frailties, the more tender you are for those of your fellow creatures.

HOLMAN E. SIR WILLIAM OSLER: TEACHER AND BIBLIOPHILE. JAMA 1969;210:2223-5.

72. *Avoid envy, be generous.*

Envy, that pain of the soul, as Plato calls it, should never for a moment afflict a man of generous instincts who has a sane outlook in life.

UNITY, PEACE, AND CONCORD, IN AEQUANIMITAS, 441.

73. *The grace of humility is a precious gift.*

And, for the sake of what it brings, this grace of humility is a precious gift. When to the sessions of sweet silent thought you summon up the remembrance of your own imperfections, the faults of your brothers will seem less grievous, and, in the quaint language of Sir Thomas Browne [1605-1682], you will "allow one eye for what is laudable in them."

TEACHER AND STUDENT, IN AEQUANIMITAS, 38-9.

74. *Respect your colleagues.*

Respect your colleagues. Know that there is no more high-minded body of men than the medical profession.

THAYER WS. OSLER THE TEACHER, IN OSLER AND OTHER PAPERS, 2.

75. *Welcome your younger colleagues.*

It is the duty of the older man to look on the younger one who settles near him not as a rival, but as a son. He will do to you just what you did to the old practitioner, when, as a young man, you started—get a good many of your cases; but if you have the sense to realize that this is inevitable, unavoidable, and the way of the world, and if you have the sense to talk over, in a friendly way, the first delicate situation that arises, the difficulties will disappear and recurrences may be made impossible.

UNITY, PEACE, AND CONCORD, IN AEQUANIMITAS, 440.

76. Never listen to tales or slander a colleague.

No sin will so easily beset you as uncharitableness towards your brother practitioner. So strong is the personal element in the practice of medicine, and so many are the wagging tongues in every parish, that evil-speaking, lying, and slandering find a shining mark in the lapses and mistakes which are inevitable in our work.

THE MASTER-WORD IN MEDICINE, IN AEQUANIMITAS, 369.

77. Never listen to a patient's criticism of another doctor.

There is only one safe rule—never listen to a patient who begins with a story about the carelessness and inefficiency of Dr. Blank. Shut him or her up with a snap, knowing full well that the same tale may be told of you a few months later. Fully half of the quarrels of physicians are fomented by the tittle-tattle of patients, and the only safeguard is not to listen.... Never believe what a patient tells you to the detriment of a brother physician even though you may think it to be true.

UNITY, PEACE AND CONCORD, IN AEQUANIMITAS, 442-3.

78. Silence is the best weapon against slander.

When we do not let the heard word die; not to listen is best, though that is not always possible, but silence is always possible, than which we have no better weapon in our armoury against evil-speaking, lying, and slandering. The bitterness is when the tale is believed and a brother's good name is involved. Then begins the worse form of ill-treatment that the practitioner receives—and at his own hands! He allows the demon of resentment to take possession of his soul, when five minutes' frank conversation might have gained a brother.

CHAUVINISM IN MEDICINE, IN AEQUANIMITAS, 287.

79. Hush the patient critical of a colleague.

Shut up at once the patient who would tell you of the faults of a professional brother. They will go to another and say the same of you. If you go with the seamy side out, the same side will be turned toward you. Go with the wooly side out and all will be well and success crown your efforts.

DR. OSLER TO STUDENTS. OKLAHOMA MED J 1900;8:53.

80. Do not judge one's colleagues by a patient's remarks.

Do not judge confreres by the reports of patients, well meaning, perhaps, but often strangely and sadly misrepresenting.

THAYER WS. OSLER THE TEACHER, IN OSLER AND OTHER PAPERS, 2.

81. Never believe a patient's criticism about a colleague.

From the day you begin practice never under any circumstances listen to a tale told to the detriment of a brother practitioner. And when any dispute or trouble does arise, go frankly, ere sunset, and talk the matter over, in which way you may gain a brother and a friend. Very easy to carry out, you may think! Far from it; there is no harder battle to fight.

THE MASTER-WORD IN MEDICINE, IN AEQUANIMITAS, 369.

82. Avoid criticizing a colleague.

Let not your ear hear the sound of your voice raised in unkind criticism or ridicule or condemnation of a brother physician.

THAYER WS. OSLER THE TEACHER, IN OSLER AND OTHER PAPERS, 2.

83. Never slander a colleague.

Never let your tongue say a slighting word of a colleague.

THAYER WS. OSLER THE TEACHER, IN OSLER AND OTHER PAPERS, 2.

84. Uncharitableness to colleagues is a pernicious vice.

The most widespread, the most pernicious of all vices, equal in its disastrous effects to impurity, much more disastrous often than intemperance, because destructive of all mental and moral nobility as are the others of bodily health, is uncharitableness—the most prevalent of modern sins, peculiarly apt to beset all of us, and the chief enemy to concord in our ranks.

UNITY, PEACE AND CONCORD, IN AEQUANIMITAS, 441.

85. Higher life is fulfilled by charity to colleagues.

The [important] lesson you may learn is the hardest of all—*that the law of the higher life is only fulfilled by love, i.e. charity.* Many a physician whose daily work is in a daily round of beneficence will say hard things and think hard things of a colleague.

THE MASTER-WORD IN MEDICINE, IN AEQUANIMITAS, 369.

86. Charity is my commandment.

I had a deep conviction to the blessings that come with unity, peace, and concord. To each of you, my brothers, to one and all, through the length and breadth of the land—I give a single word as my parting commandment...charity.

HOLMAN E. SIR WILLIAM OSLER: TEACHER AND BIBLIOPHILE. JAMA 1969;210:2223-5.

87. Foster generosity.

May I say a word on the art of giving? The essence is contained in the well-known sentence, "let every man do according as he is disposed in his heart, not grudgingly or of necessity." Subscriptions to a cause which is for the benefit of the entire profession should truly be given as a man is disposed in his heart, not in his pocket, and assuredly not of necessity, but as a duty, even as a privilege, and as a pleasure. Some of us, the younger men, cannot give. The days of travail and distress are not yet over, and to give would be wrong. It is sufficient for such to have the wish to give; the elder brothers will bear your share; only be sure to foster those generous impulses, which are apt to be intense in direct proportion to the emptiness of your purse.

THE FUNCTIONS OF A STATE FACULTY. MARYLAND MED J 1897;37:73-7.

88. Osler apologizes for unwitting offenses.

It may be that in the hurry and bustle of a busy life I have given offense to some—who can avoid it? Unwittingly I may have shot an arrow o'er the house and hurt a brother—if so, I am sorry and I ask his pardon. So far as I can read my heart I leave you in charity with all.

UNITY, PEACE AND CONCORD. MARYLAND MED J 1905;48:412-22.

89. Say nothing and look wise.

Look wise, say nothing, and grunt. Speech was given to conceal thought.

BEAN WB. SIR WILLIAM OSLER: APHORISMS, 130.

90. Keep your mouth shut.

Printed in your remembrance, written as headlines on the tablets of your chatelaines [the lady of a castle], I would have two maxims: "I will keep my mouth shut as it were with a bridle," and "If thou hast heard a word let it die with thee." Taciturnity, a discreet silence, is a virtue little cultivated in these garrulous days when the chatter of the bander-log [from *The Jungle Book* by Rudyard Kipling (1865-1936). The bander-log were monkeys.] is everywhere about us, when, as some one has remarked, speech has taken the place of thought.

NURSE AND PATIENT, IN AEQUANIMITAS, 153.

91. *Silence is powerful.*

Silence is a powerful weapon.

THAYER WS. OSLER THE TEACHER, IN OSLER AND OTHER PAPERS, 2.

92. *Beware of words.*

Beware of words—they are dangerous things. They change colour like the chameleon, and they return like a boomerang.

THAYER WS. OSLER THE TEACHER, IN OSLER AND OTHER PAPERS, 3.

93. *Speak only when you have something to say.*

But in your relation with the profession and with the public, in everything that pertains to medicine, consider the virtues of taciturnity. Look out. Speak only when you have something to say. Commit yourself only when you can and must. And when you speak, assert only that which you know.

THAYER WS. OSLER THE TEACHER, IN OSLER AND OTHER PAPERS, 3.

94. *The public, nurses, and physicians should be discreet.*

With the growth of one abominable practice [idle chatter]...I refer to the habit of openly discussing ailments which should never be mentioned. Doubtless it is in a measure the result of the disgusting publicity in which we live, and to the pernicious habit of allowing the filth of the gutters as purveyed in the newspapers to pollute the stream of our daily lives. This open talk about personal maladies is an atrocious breach of good manners.... We doctors are great sinners in this manner, and among ourselves and with the laity are much too fond of "talking shop."

NURSE AND PATIENT, IN AEQUANIMITAS, 153-4.

95. Nurses should be discreet about patients.

To talk of disease [in a patient] is a sort of Arabian Nights' entertainment to which no discreet nurse will lend her talents.

NURSING AND PATIENT, IN AEQUANIMITAS, 153.

96. Do not breach privacy.

Never under any circumstances tell moving stories of cases, never for a moment divulge what has passed within the house of another patient, utter no word about your past record as a nurse in connection with cases,—nothing on any of these subjects should ever pass your lips.

COMMENCEMENT ADDRESS TO THE NURSES OF THE JOHNS HOPKINS TRAINING SCHOOL,
MAY 7, 1913. JOHNS HOPKINS HOSP NURSES ALUM MAG 1913;12:72-81.

97. The press can be dangerous.

In the life of every successful physician there comes the temptation to toy with the Delilah of the press—daily and otherwise. There are times when she may be courted with satisfaction, but beware! sooner or later she is sure to play the harlot, and has left many a man shorn of his strength, viz, the confidence of his professional brethren.

INTERNAL MEDICINE AS A VOCATION, IN AEQUANIMITAS, 144.

98. The physician-patient relationship requires confidentiality.

It is time that honorable physicians set their faces against this ever-increasing habit of furnishing representatives of the press with details which satisfy no public purpose, but which simply minister to the morbid longings of a prurient and gossip-loving public. In this irreverent generation, the almost sacred character of the relation of the physician and patient has come to be lightly regarded, and the modern reporter, with an assurance strengthened by success, asks for, and expects to obtain, information of the most private nature. That he should so often procure it, is a sad evidence of degeneracy in the profession, and of the neglect of that most important section of the Hippocratic oath.

DEMENTIA PARALYTICA AND SYPHILIS. MED NEWS [PHILADELPHIA] 1886;48:40-1.

99. Doubt the press.

Believe nothing that you see in the newspapers—they have done more to create dissatisfaction than all other agencies. If you see anything in them that you know is true, begin to doubt it at once.

BEAN WB. SIR WILLIAM OSLER: APHORISMS, 64.

Time Management and Work Ethic

100. Success leaves no time to relax.

The stress of commercial battle presses sore on the finer spirits as success means absorption, such intense absorption, in the work of the day that there is not a moment left for "the things that pertain to his peace."

BURROWINGS OF A BOOK-WORM, EGERTON YORRICK DAVIS JR., GOLDEN, R. THE
WORKS OF EGERTON YORRICK DAVIS, MD/SIR WILLIAM OSLER'S ALTER EGO,
MONTREAL:OSLER LIBRARY, 1999.

101. Past success predicts future success.

In the race upon which you enter today, the success or failure, as the case may be, will depend very much on the life which is now behind you. It has passed by but its effects for good or evil remain. If you have been idle and wasteful of your time at school it will be hard to acquire industrious habits here.

UNPUBLISHED DRAFT OF AN ADDRESS TO MEDICAL STUDENTS AT THE UNIVERSITY OF PENNSYLVANIA, 1885. PUBLISHED PRIVATELY BY THE OSLER LIBRARY, MCGILL UNIVERSITY, MONTREAL, 2006.

102. Resolve not to waste time.

Bury the past and start afresh today with the firm resolve to waste not an hour of the short and precious time which is before you.

UNPUBLISHED DRAFT OF AN ADDRESS TO MEDICAL STUDENTS AT THE UNIVERSITY OF PENNSYLVANIA, 1885. PUBLISHED PRIVATELY BY THE OSLER LIBRARY, MCGILL UNIVERSITY, MONTREAL, 2006.

103. Learn to be thorough first.

To those of you who are beginning I would say, start slowly, take one thing at a time, and do not leave it until you have conquered a few facts regarding it. Learn the lesson of thoroughness at the outset or you are apt not [to] learn it at all.

UNPUBLISHED DRAFT OF AN ADDRESS TO MEDICAL STUDENTS AT THE UNIVERSITY OF PENNSYLVANIA, 1885. PUBLISHED PRIVATELY BY THE OSLER LIBRARY, MCGILL UNIVERSITY, MONTREAL, 2006.

104. Absorb knowledge with small, frequent helpings.

Understand clearly that you cannot absorb knowledge continuously in large quantities, any more than you can take an indefinite amount of food. You will find at first that your mental stomach can neither hold nor digest much, but the secret of success of intellectual assimilation lies in taking small but often repeated portions of knowledge.

UNPUBLISHED DRAFT OF AN ADDRESS TO MEDICAL STUDENTS AT THE UNIVERSITY OF
PENNSYLVANIA, 1885. PUBLISHED PRIVATELY BY THE OSLER LIBRARY, MCGILL
UNIVERSITY, MONTREAL, 2006.

105. The master-word in medicine is work.

I propose to tell you the secret of life as I have seen the game played, and as I have tried to play it myself.... Though a little one, the master-word looms large in meaning. It is the open sesame to every portal, the great equalizer in the world, the true philosopher's stone, which transmutes all the base metal of humanity into gold. The stupid man among you it will make bright, the bright man brilliant, and the brilliant student steady. With the magic word in your heart all things are possible, and without it all study is vanity and vexation. The miracles of life are with it; the blind see by touch, the deaf hear with eyes, the dumb speak with fingers. To the youth it brings hope, to the middle-aged confidence, to the aged repose. True balm of hurt minds, in its presence the heart of the sorrowful is lightened and consoled. It is directly responsible for all advances in medicine during the past twenty-five centuries.... And the master-word is *Work*, a little one, as I have said, but fraught with momentous sequences if you can but write it on the tablets of your hearts, and bind it upon your foreheads.

THE MASTER-WORD IN MEDICINE, IN AEQUANIMITAS, 356-7.

106. Steady work is the talisman of life.

Steady work...gives a man a sane outlook on the world. No corrective [is] so valuable to the weariness, the fever, and the fret that are so apt to wring the heart of the young. This is the talisman, as George Herbert [(1593-1633), English metaphysical poet] says,

The famous stone / That turneth all to gold... [from "The Elixir"]

and with which, to the eternally recurring question, What is Life? you answer, I do not think—I act it; the only philosophy that brings you in contact with its real values and enables you to grasp its hidden meaning. Over the Slough of Despond, past Doubting Castle and Giant Despair, with this talisman you may reach the Delectable Mountains, and those Shepherds of the Mind—Knowledge, Experience, Watchful, and Sincere [referring to the landmarks in *The Pilgrim's Progress* by John Bunyan (1628-1688)].

A WAY OF LIFE, IN A WAY OF LIFE, 247.

107. Hard work will triumph over genius.

Let such believe the truth that fair average abilities, well used, often carry their owner above the heads of abler men—the genius rarely makes a successful practitioner; but the careful hard-working student who feels that he must grind up his subject with plodding pains before he can make it a part of himself, and who acts on this impression, develops the elements of life-long success during his academic course.

INTRODUCTORY LECTURE, 17.

108. Thoroughness is a difficult habit to acquire.

Thoroughness is the most difficult habit to acquire, but it is the pearl of great price, worth all the worry and trouble of the search. The dilettante lives an easy, butterfly life, knowing nothing of the toil and labour with which the treasures of knowledge are dug out of the past, or wrung by patient research in the laboratories.

THE STUDENT LIFE, IN AEQUANIMITAS, 401.

109. Punctuality is a prime essential for a physician.

Punctuality is the prime essential of a physician—if invariably on time he will succeed even in the face of professional mediocrity.

HOLMAN E. SIR WILLIAM OSLER: TEACHER AND BIBLIOPHILE. JAMA 1969;210:2223-5.

110. The virtue of method is a secret to success.

Ask of any active business man or a leader in a profession the secret which enables him to accomplish much work, and he will reply in one word, *system;* or as I shall term it, the *Virtue of Method,* the harness without which only the horses of genius travel.

TEACHER AND STUDENT, IN AEQUANIMITAS, 34.

111. Appreciate the value of system.

Take away with you a profound conviction of the value of system in your work.

THE MASTER-WORD IN MEDICINE, IN AEQUANIMITAS, 361.

112. Study by system.

Thus faithfully followed day by day system may become at last engrained in the most shiftless nature, and at the end of a semester a youth of moderate ability may find himself far in advance of the student who works spasmodically, and trusts to *cramming.*

TEACHER AND STUDENT, IN AEQUANIMITAS, 34.

113. Cultivate systematic habits.

How can you take the greatest possible advantage of your capacities with the least possible strain? By cultivating system. I say cultivating advisedly, since some of you will find the acquisition of systematic habits very hard.

THE MASTER-WORD IN MEDICINE, IN AEQUANIMITAS, 360.

114. Cultivate a method of studying.

Let me add a word of advice on the method of studying. The secret of successful working lies in the systematic arrangement of what you have to do, and in the methodical performance of it. With all of you this is possible, for few disturbing elements exist in the student's life to interrupt the allotted duty which each hour of the day should possess. Make out, each one for himself, a time-table, with the hours of lecture, study, and recreation, and follow closely and conscientiously the programme there indicated. I know of no better way to accomplish a large amount of work, and it saves the mental worry and anxiety which will surely haunt you if your tasks are done in an irregular and desultory way.

INTRODUCTORY LECTURE, 11.

115. Cultivate the power of concentration.

Let each hour of the day have its allotted duty, and cultivate that power of concentration which grows with its exercise, so that the attention neither flags nor wavers, but settles with a bull-dog tenacity on the subject before you. Constant repetition makes a good habit fit easily in your mind, and by the end of the session you may have gained that most precious of all knowledge—the power of work.

THE MASTER-WORD IN MEDICINE, IN AEQUANIMITAS, 361.

116. Control the mind as a habit.

Control of the mind as a working machine, the adaptation in it of habit, so that its action becomes almost as automatic as walking, is the end of education—and yet how rarely reached! It can be accomplished with deliberation and repose, never with hurry and worry. Realize how much time there is, how long the day is. Realize that you have sixteen waking hours, three or four of which at least should be devoted to making a silent conquest of your mental machinery.

A WAY OF LIFE, IN A WAY OF LIFE, 245-6.

117. Take routine into your daily life.

I appeal to the freshmen especially, because you to-day make a beginning, and your future career depends very much upon the habits you will form during this session. To follow the routine of the classes is easy enough, but to take routine into every part of your daily life is a hard task.

THE MASTER-WORD IN MEDICINE, IN AEQUANIMITAS, 361.

118. Do what lies clearly at hand.

Throw away...all ambition beyond that of doing the day's work well. The travelers on the road to success live in the present, heedless of taking thought for the morrow, having been able at some time, and in some form or other, to receive into their heart of hearts this maxim of the Sage of Chelsea [Thomas Carlyle (1795-1881), Scottish historian and critic]: Your business is "not to see what lies dimly at a distance, but to do what lies clearly at hand."

THE ARMY SURGEON, IN AEQUANIMITAS, 104.

119. Do first what has to be done.

Think not of the amount to be accomplished, the difficulties to be overcome, or the end to be attained, but set earnestly at the little task at your elbow, letting that be sufficient for the day.

INTRODUCTORY LECTURE, 11.

120. Live in the present.

As to your method of work, I have a single bit of advice, which I give with the earnest conviction of its paramount influence in any success which may have attended my efforts in life—*Take therefore no thought for the morrow* [from the Sermon on the Mount, Matthew 6:34]. Live neither in the past nor in the future, but let each day's work absorb your entire energies, and satisfy your widest ambition.

AFTER TWENTY-FIVE YEARS, IN AEQUANIMITAS, 204.

121. Shut off the past.

Shut off the past! Let the dead past bury its dead. So easy to say, so hard to realize! The truth is, the past haunts us like a shadow. To disregard it is not easy.

A WAY OF LIFE, IN A WAY OF LIFE, 241.

122. The future is today.

The load of to-morrow, added to that of yesterday, carried to-day makes the strongest falter. Shut off the future as tightly as the past. No dreams, no visions, no delicious fantasies, no castles in the air, with which, as the old song so truly says, "hearts are broken, heads are turned." To youth, we are told, belongs the future, but the wretched to-morrow that so plagues some of us has no certainty, except through to-day. Who can tell what a day may bring forth?…The future is to-day—there is no to-morrow! The day of a man's salvation is *now*—the life of the present, of to-day, lived earnestly, intently, without a forward-looking thought, is the only insurance for the future. Let the limit of your horizon be a twenty-four-hour circle.

A WAY OF LIFE, IN A WAY OF LIFE, 242.

123. Live in day-tight compartments.

The quiet life in day-tight compartments will help you to bear your own and others' burdens with a light heart. Pay no heed to the Batrachians [frogs and toads] who sit croaking idly by the stream. Life is a straight, plain business, and the way is clear, blazed for you by generations of strong men, into whose labours you enter and whose ideals must be your inspiration.

A WAY OF LIFE, IN A WAY OF LIFE, 249.

124. Learn to live one day at a time.

The way of life that I preach is a habit to be acquired gradually by long and steady repetition. It is the practice of living for the day only, and for the day's work, *Life in day-tight compartments.*

A WAY OF LIFE, IN A WAY OF LIFE, 239.

125. Map out your day.

Do not underestimate the difficulty you will have in wringing from your reluctant selves the stern determination to exact the uttermost minute on your schedule. Do not get too interested in one study at the expense of another, but so map out your day that due allowance is given to each. Only in this way can the average student get the best that he can out of his capacities. And it is worth all the pains and trouble he can possibly take for the ultimate gain—if he can reach his doctorate with system so ingrained that it has become an integral part of his being.

THE MASTER-WORD IN MEDICINE, IN AEQUANIMITAS, 361-2.

126. Do your duty day by day.

You will not only be better, but happier men, if you endeavour to do your duty day by day, not from self interest, not from any outside aim however high, but simply because it is right, content to let the reward come when it will.

INTRODUCTORY LECTURE, 19.

127. Success is doing the day's work well.

I started in life—I may as well own up and admit—with just an ordinary everyday stock of brains. In my schooldays I was much more bent upon mischief than upon books—I say it with regret now—but as soon as I got interested in medicine I had only the single idea of doing the day's work faithfully and honestly, as well as I could, and I do believe that if I have had any measure of success at all, it has been solely and wholly in doing the day's work that was before me just as actively and just as energetically and just as well as was in my power.

ADDRESS TO THE STUDENTS OF THE ALBANY MEDICAL COLLEGE. ALBANY MED ANN
1899;20:307-9.

128. Find peace by focusing on the present.

As a patient with double vision from some transient unequal action of the muscles of the eye finds magical relief from well-adjusted glasses, so, returning to the clear binocular vision of to-day, the over-anxious student finds peace when he looks neither backward to the past nor forward to the future.

A WAY OF LIFE, IN A WAY OF LIFE, 240.

129. Renew yourself daily.

Many a man is handicapped in his course by a cursed combination of retro- and intro-spection, the mistakes of yesterday paralysing the efforts of to-day, the worries of the past hugged to his destruction, and the worm Regret allowed to canker the very heart of his life. To die daily, after the manner of St. Paul, ensures the resurrection of a new man, who makes each day the epitome of a life.

A WAY OF LIFE, IN A WAY OF LIFE, 242.

130. Dodge the bore.

Save the fleeting minute; do not stop by the way. Learn gracefully to dodge the bore. Strike first and quickly, and before he has recovered from the blow, be gone; 'tis the only way...

THAYER WS. OSLER THE TEACHER, IN OSLER AND OTHER PAPERS, 4.

2

The Art and Practice
of Medicine

- → The Art of Medicine and Counseling the
  Patient

- → The Practice of Medicine

- → Financial and Material Interests of Practice

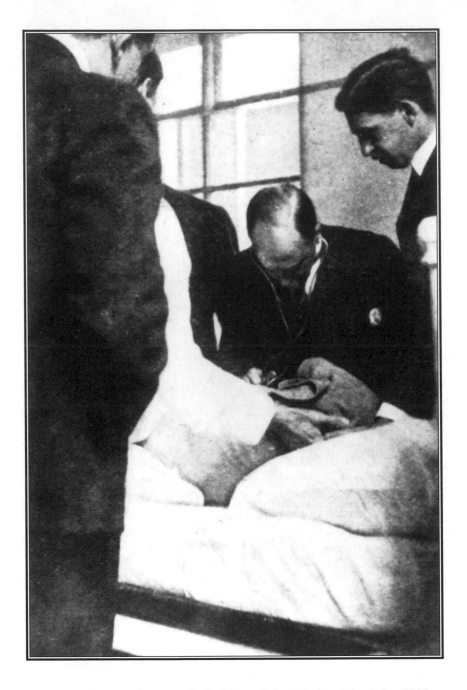

William Osler auscultating at the bedside at Johns Hopkins Hospital in 1903.
(Courtesy of the Alan Mason Chesney Medical Archives
of the Johns Hopkins Medical Institutions.)

The Art and Practice of Medicine

The Art of Medicine and Counseling the Patient

131. Be sympathetic.

The kindly word, the cheerful greeting, the sympathetic look, [though] trivial they may seem, help to brighten the paths of the poor sufferers and are often as "oil and wine" to the bruised spirits entrusted to our care.

UNPUBLISHED DRAFT OF AN ADDRESS TO MEDICAL STUDENTS AT THE UNIVERSITY OF PENNSYLVANIA, 1885. PUBLISHED PRIVATELY BY THE OSLER LIBRARY, MCGILL UNIVERSITY, MONTREAL, 2006.

132. Be kind and gentle.

Kindliness of disposition and gentleness of manners are qualities essential in a practitioner. If they do not exist naturally, they are virtues which must be cultivated if not be assumed. The rough voice, the hard sharp answer, and the blunt manner are as much out of place in the hospital ward as "any lady's boudoir."

UNPUBLISHED DRAFT OF AN ADDRESS TO MEDICAL STUDENTS AT THE UNIVERSITY OF PENNSYLVANIA, 1885. PUBLISHED PRIVATELY BY THE OSLER LIBRARY, MCGILL UNIVERSITY, MONTREAL, 2006.

133. *Care for the patient, not the disease.*

Care more particularly for the individual patient than for the special features of the disease.

ADDRESS TO THE STUDENTS OF THE ALBANY MEDICAL COLLEGE. ALBANY MED ANN 1899;20:307-9.

134. *Each patient is different.*

Our study is man, as the subject of accidents or disease. Were he always, inside and outside, cast in the same mould, instead of differing from his fellow man as much in constitution and in his reaction to stimulus as in feature, we should ere this have reached some settled principles in our art.

TEACHER AND STUDENT, IN AEQUANIMITAS, 35.

135. *Empathize with the patient.*

The motto of each of you as you undertake the examination and treatment of a case should be "put yourself in his place." Realize, so far as you can, the mental state of the patient, enter into his feelings. . . . Scan gently his faults. The kindly word, the cheerful greeting, the sympathetic look.

PENFIELD W. NEUROLOGY IN CANADA AND THE OSLER CENTENNIAL. CAN MED ASSOC J 1949;61:69-73.

136. *Practice the golden rule.*

In some of us the ceaseless panorama of suffering tends to dull that fine edge of sympathy with which we started. . . . Against this benumbing influence, we physicians and nurses, the immediate agents of the Trust, have but one enduring corrective—the practice towards patients of the Golden Rule of Humanity as announced by Confucius [6th century B.C. Chinese philosopher]: "What you do not like when done to yourself, do not do to others."

NURSE AND PATIENT, IN AEQUANIMITAS, 159.

137. *Love in order to serve medicine.*

To serve the art of medicine as it should be served, one must love his fellow man.

THE EVOLUTION OF INTERNAL MEDICINE. IN MODERN MEDICINE: ITS THEORY AND ITS PRACTICE. PHILADELPHIA: LEA BROTHERS, 1907:34.

138. *Medicine exercises your heart and your head.*

The practice of medicine is an art, not a trade; a calling, not a business; a calling in which your heart will be exercised equally with your head.

THE MASTER-WORD IN MEDICINE, IN AEQUANIMITAS, 368.

139. *The best part of your work will be your influence and comfort.*

Often the best part of your work will have nothing to do with potions and powders, but with the exercise of an influence of the strong upon the weak, of the righteous upon the wicked, of the wise upon the foolish. To you, as the trusted family counsellor, the father will come with his anxieties, the mother with her hidden grief, the daughter with her trials, and the son with his follies. Fully one-third of the work you do will be entered in other books than yours. Courage and cheerfulness will not only carry you over the rough places of life, but will enable you to bring comfort and help to the weak-hearted and will console you in the sad hours when, like Uncle Toby [a compassionate character in *Tristram Shandy* by Laurence Sterne (1713-1768)], you have "to whistle that you may not weep."

THE MASTER-WORD IN MEDICINE, IN AEQUANIMITAS, 368-9.

140. Tolerate uncertainty.

A distressing feature in the life which you are about to enter, a feature which will press hardly upon the finer spirits among you and ruffle their equanimity, is the uncertainty which pertains not alone to our science and art, but to the very hopes and fears which make us men. In seeking absolute truth we aim at the unattainable, and must be content with finding broken portions.

AEQUANIMITAS, IN AEQUANIMITAS, 6-7.

141. Errors cannot be avoided.

Errors in judgment must occur in the practice of an art which consists largely of balancing probabilities.

TEACHER AND STUDENT, IN AEQUANIMITAS, 38.

142. Medicine is an art of probability.

Medicine is a science of uncertainty and an art of probability.

BEAN WB. SIR WILLIAM OSLER: APHORISMS, 129.

143. Medicine is an art.

The practice of medicine is an art, based on science.

TEACHER AND STUDENT, IN AEQUANIMITAS, 34.

144. The art of medicine is a servant to science.

The art [of medicine] is very apt to outrun or override the science, and play the master where the true role is that of the servant.

THE TREATMENT OF DISEASE. CAN LANCET 1909;42:899-912.

145. The greatest art is concealment of art.

The greatest art is in the concealment of art, and I may say that we of the medical profession excel in this respect.

TEACHING AND THINKING, IN AEQUANIMITAS, 118.

146. The art of medicine cannot be replaced.

It is much harder to acquire the art than the science. . . . There is still virtue, believe me, in that "long unlovely street" [Harley Street in London where private physicians and surgeons practice], and the old art cannot possibly be replaced by, but must be absorbed in, the new science.

THE RESERVES OF LIFE. ST. MARY'S HOSP GAZ 1907;13:95-8.

147. The art of the practice of medicine is learned by experience.

The art of the practice of medicine is to be learned only by experience; 'tis not an inheritance; it cannot be revealed. Learn to see, learn to hear, learn to feel, learn to smell, and know that by practice alone can you become expert.

THAYER WS. OSLER THE TEACHER, IN OSLER AND OTHER PAPERS, 1.

148. There is no discredit to say "perhaps."

The practitioner too often gets into a habit of mind which resents the thought that opinion, not full knowledge, must be his stay and prop.

There is no discredit, though there is at times much discomfort, in this everlasting *perhaps* with which we have to preface so much connected with the practice of our art. It is, as I said, inherent in the subject.

ON THE EDUCATIONAL VALUE OF THE MEDICAL SOCIETY, IN AEQUANIMITAS, 332

149. Gain the patient's confidence.

Once gain the confidence of a patient and inspire him with hope, and the battle is half won.

THE RESERVES OF LIFE. ST. MARY'S HOSP GAZ 1907;13:95-8.

150. Take a lady's hand.

Taking a lady's hand gives her confidence in her physician.

BEAN WB. SIR WILLIAM OSLER: APHORISMS, 130.

151. Telling a patient that he is past hope is hard.

A disease itself may be incurable and the best we can do is to relieve symptoms and to make the patient comfortable. . . . It is a hard matter and really not often necessary (since nature usually does it quietly and in good time) to tell a patient that he is past all hope. As Sir Thomas Browne [1605-1682] says: "It is the hardest stone you can throw at a man to tell him that he is at the end of his tether;" [from *Urn-Burial;* or *Hydriotaphia*] and yet, put in the right way to an intelligent man it is not always cruel.

THE TREATMENT OF DISEASE. CAN LANCET 1909;42:899-912.

152. Do not take hope away from the patient.

What is your duty in the matter of telling a patient that he is probably the subject of an incurable disease? . . . One thing is certain; it is not for you to don the black cap, and, assuming the judicial function, take hope from any patient—"hope that comes to all."

LECTURES ON ANGINA PECTORIS AND ALLIED STATES, 142.

The Practice of Medicine

153. Recognize the poetry of the commonplace.

Nothing will sustain you more potently than the power to recognize in your humdrum routine, as perhaps it may be thought, the true poetry of life—the poetry of the commonplace, of the ordinary man, of the plain, toil-worn woman, with their loves and their joys, their sorrows and their griefs.

THE STUDENT LIFE, IN AEQUANIMITAS, 404-5.

154. The practice of medicine is what you make it.

To each one of you the practice of medicine will be very much as you make it—to one a worry, a care, a perpetual annoyance; to another, a daily joy and a life of as much happiness and usefulness as can well fall to the lot of man.

THE STUDENT LIFE, IN AEQUANIMITAS, 423.

155. Appreciate the comic side of life.

The comedy, too, of life will be spread before you, and nobody laughs more often than the doctor at the pranks Puck plays upon the Titanias and the Bottoms [referring to Shakespeare's (1564-1616) *A Midsummer Night's Dream*] among his patients. The humorous side is really almost as frequently turned towards him as the tragic. Lift up one hand to heaven and thank your stars if they have given you the proper sense to enable you to appreciate the inconceivably droll situations in which we catch our fellow creatures.

THE STUDENT LIFE, IN AEQUANIMITAS, 405.

156. Don't take yourself or others too seriously.

But whatever you do, take neither yourselves nor your fellow-creatures too seriously. There is tragedy enough in our daily routine, but there is room too for a keen sense of the absurdities and incongruities of life, and in the shifting panorama no one sees better than the doctor the perennial sameness of men's ways.

THE RESERVES OF LIFE. ST. MARY'S HOSP GAZ 1907;13:95-8.

157. Make allowances for the weaknesses of patients.

Our work is an incessant collection of evidence, weighing of evidence, and judging upon the evidence, and we have to learn early to make large allowances for our own frailty, and still larger for the weaknesses, often involuntary, of our patients.

THE EVOLUTION OF INTERNAL MEDICINE. IN MODERN MEDICINE: ITS THEORY AND PRACTICE. PHILADELPHIA: LEA BROTHERS, 1907:31.

158. The practice of medicine can be a testy business.

It must be confessed that the practice of medicine among our fellow creatures is often a testy and choleric business.

CHAUVINISM IN MEDICINE, IN AEQUANIMITAS, 286-7.

159. Cultivate your hearts and your heads.

Be careful when you get into practice to cultivate equally well your hearts and your heads.

ADDRESS TO THE STUDENTS OF THE ALBANY MEDICAL COLLEGE. ALBANY MED ANN 1899;20:307-9.

160. A physician needs a clear head and kind heart.

The physician needs a clear head and a kind heart; his work is arduous and complex, requiring the exercise of the very highest faculties of the mind, while constantly appealing to the emotions and finer feelings.

TEACHING AND THINKING, IN AEQUANIMITAS, 126.

161. The practice of medicine is controlled by the heart.

As the practice of medicine is not a business and can never be one, the education of the heart—the moral side of the man—must keep pace with the education of the head. Our fellow creatures cannot be dealt with as man deals in corn and coal; "the human heart by which we live" [from *Ode (Intimations of Immortality from Recollections of Early Childhood)* by William Wordsworth (1770-1850)] must control our professional relations. After all, the personal equation has most to do with success or failure in medicine, and in the trials of life the fire which strengthens and tempers the metal of one may soften and ruin another.

ON THE EDUCATIONAL VALUE OF THE MEDICAL SOCIETY, IN AEQUANIMITAS, 333.

162. The physician's heart is the most important aspect of practice.

Of the three factors in practice, heart, head, and pocket, to our credit, be it said, the first named is most potent.

PENFIELD W. NEUROLOGY IN CANADA AND THE OSLER CENTENNIAL. CAN MED ASSOC J 1949;61:69-73.

163. We are here to make the lives of others happier.

The practitioner of medicine . . . we are here not to get all we can out of life for ourselves, but to try to make the lives of others happier.

THE MASTER-WORD IN MEDICINE, IN AEQUANIMITAS, 368.

164. Treat your fellow man kindly.

Individually, man, the unit, the microcosm, is fast bound in chains of atavism, inheriting legacies of feeble will and strong desires, taints of blood and brain. What wonder, then, that many, sore let and hindered in running the race, fall by the way, and need a shelter in which to recruit or to die, a hospital, in which there shall be no harsh comments on conduct, but only, so far as is possible, love and peace and rest? Here, we learn to scan gently our brother man, judging not, asking no questions, but meting out to all alike a hospitality worthy of the *Hôtel Dieu,* and deeming ourselves honoured in being allowed to act as its dispensers.

DOCTOR AND NURSE, IN AEQUANIMITAS, 17.

165. Our work is relieved by the devotion of our patients.

Amid an eternal heritage of sorrow and suffering our work is laid, and this eternal note of sadness would be insupportable if the daily tragedies were not relieved by the spectacle of the heroism and devotion displayed by the actors.

THE STUDENT LIFE, IN AEQUANIMITAS, 404.

166. Give the time needed for the patient.

The clinician who keeps one eye on his watch while in the wards is rarely successful.

ON THE INFLUENCE OF A HOSPITAL UPON THE MEDICAL PROFESSION OF A COMMUNITY. ALBANY MED ANN 1901;22:1-11.

167. Medical practice is inefficient.

The average physician wastes fifty to sixty per cent of his time in going from place to place or in the repetition of uninstructive details of practice.

GWYN N. THE EARLY LIFE OF SIR WILLIAM OSLER. IN ABBOTT ME (ED). SIR WILLIAM
OSLER MEMORIAL NUMBER. BULLETIN NO. IX OF THE INTERNATIONAL ASSOCIATION OF
MEDICAL MUSEUMS AND JOURNAL OF TECHNICAL METHODS. MONTREAL: PRIVATELY
PRINTED, 1926:143.

168. Derive power from the faithfulness of small things.

Faithfulness in the day of small things will insensibly widen your powers, correct your faculties; and, in moments of despondency, comfort may be derived from a knowledge that some of the best work of the profession has come from men whose clinical field was limited but well-tilled.

THE ARMY SURGEON, IN AEQUANIMITAS, 105.

169. The patient of all ages and all problems is the subject of our study and care.

Man, with all his mental and bodily anomalies and diseases—the machine in order, the machine in disorder, and the business yours to put it to rights. Through all the phases of its career this most complicated mechanism of this wonderful world will be the subject of our study and of your care—the naked, new-born infant, the artless child, the lad and the lassie just aware of the tree of knowledge overhead, the strong man in the pride of life, the woman with the benediction of maternity on her brow, and the aged, peaceful in the contemplation of the past.

THE STUDENT LIFE, IN AEQUANIMITAS, 404.

170. Physicians have several challenges.

The physician's challenge is the curing of disease, educating the people in the laws of health, and preventing the spread of plagues and pestilences.

BEAN WB. SIR WILLIAM OSLER: APHORISMS, 63.

171. These are our ambitions.

To wrest from nature the secrets which have perplexed philosophers in all ages, to track to their sources the causes of disease, to correlate the vast stores of knowledge, that they may be quickly available for the prevention and cure of disease—these are our ambitions.

CHAUVINISM IN MEDICINE, IN AEQUANIMITAS, 267.

172. The duties of the physician are several.

We know more and enjoy larger opportunities and with them have greater responsibilities, but could Hippocrates return he would find no change in those essential duties in which he is still our great exemplar. They are four: so to study our cases as to acquire facility in the art of diagnosis, which must everywhere precede the rational treatment of disease; so to grow in clinical judgement that we may learn to appreciate the relative value of the symptoms and physical signs, and give to the patient and his friends a forecast or prognosis; so to conduct the treatment that the patient may be restored to health at the earliest possible period, or, failing that, be given the greatest possible measure of relief, whether by drugs, the action of which he should carefully study, so as to have a strong and abiding faith in those which have been tried and not found wanting, by diet, by exercise, or by all the physical means available, and often by the exercise of his own strong personality; and lastly, so to arrange sanitary and hygienic measures that, wherever possible, disease may be prevented.

THE EVOLUTION OF INTERNAL MEDICINE. IN MODERN MEDICINE: ITS THEORY AND PRACTICE. PHILADELPHIA: LEA BROTHERS, 1907:34.

173. Live to our threefold capacity.

In his character as a physician a man has a threefold relation: with the public, with the profession and with himself. Not one of us in all, only a few of us in some of these diverse relations, live up to our full capacity.

DR. JOHNSTON AS A PHYSICIAN. WASHINGTON MED ANN 1902;1:158-61.

174. The uncertainties of medicine make us despair.

At times, and in degrees differing with our temperaments, there come upon us bouts of depression, when we feel that the battle has been lost, and that to fight longer is not worth the effort, periods when, amid the weariness, the fever and the fret of daily practice, things have gone against us; we have been misunderstood by patients, our motives have been wrongly interpreted, and smitten perhaps in the house of our friends, the worries of heart to which we doctors are so subject make us feel bitterly the uncertainties of medicine as a profession, and at times make us despair of its future.

ELISHA BARTLETT, IN AN ALABAMA STUDENT, 137-8.

175. Perplexity of soul will be your lot.

As perplexity of soul will be your lot and portion, accept the situation with a good grace. The hopes and fears which make us men are inseparable, and this wine-press of Doubt each of you must tread alone. It is a trouble from which no man may deliver his brother or make agreement with another for him.

SCIENCE AND IMMORTALITY, 42.

176. Happiness lies in a vocation that satisfies the soul.

Practically there should be for each of you a busy, useful, and happy life; more you cannot expect; a greater blessing the world cannot bestow. Busy you will certainly be, as the demand is great. . . . Useful your lives must be, as you will care for those who cannot care for themselves. . . . And happy lives shall be yours, because busy and useful; having been initiated into the great secret—that happiness lies in the absorption in some vocation which satisfies the soul; that we are here to add what we can *to*, not to get what we can *from*, life.

DOCTOR AND NURSE, IN AEQUANIMITAS, 19.

177. Medicine is all-absorbing.

The medical profession in every country has produced men of affairs of the first rank, men who have risen high in the councils of nations, but with scarcely an exception the practice of medicine has not been compatible with such duties. So absorbing are the cares of the general practitioner or the successful consultant, that he has but little time to mingle in outside affairs, and the few who enter public life do so with many backward glances at the consulting-room, and with well-grounded forebodings of disaster to professional work.

WILLIAM PEPPER, IN AN ALABAMA STUDENT, 224-5.

178. The plain language of healing is the more useful.

And from the standpoint of medicine as an art for the prevention and cure of disease, the man who translates the hieroglyphics of science into the plain language of healing is certainly the more useful.

TEACHER AND STUDENT, IN AEQUANIMITAS, 30.

179. The practice of medicine requires knowledge of basic science.

A man cannot become a competent surgeon without a full knowledge of human anatomy and physiology, and the physician without physiology and chemistry flounders along in an aimless fashion, never able to gain any accurate conception of disease, practising a sort of popgun pharmacy, hitting now the malady and again the patient, he himself not knowing which.

TEACHING AND THINKING, IN AEQUANIMITAS, 121.

180. A physician can pursue scientific research or medical practice.

There are two avenues to success in practice; the one a broad and much travelled road, the *via publica*, smooth and easy, well paved, without ruts, along which the average doctor can jog along behind common-sense (medical) and civility, by far the best team of their kind; the other, the *via medica* a straight and narrow way, but very rough, along which many start, full of life, driving, not a team but science, in single harness.

ON THE INFLUENCE OF A HOSPITAL UPON THE MEDICAL PROFESSION OF A COMMUNITY.
ALBANY MED ANN 1901;22:1-11.

181. Add your reports to medical knowledge.

Let it be also an ambition to add your mite [contribution] to the store of medical knowledge. Every one can do something; and the routine of general practice affords many cases worth reporting or commenting upon.

VALEDICTORY ADDRESS TO THE GRADUATES IN MEDICINE AND SURGERY, McGILL
UNIVERSITY. CAN MED SURG J 1874-75;3:433-42.

182. Successful physicians make fewer mistakes.

The best doctor, like the successful general, is the one who makes the fewest mistakes.

THE PATHOLOGICAL INSTITUTE OF A GENERAL HOSPITAL. GLASGOW MED J
1911;76:321-33.

183. Successful doctors may practice poor medicine.

It is only too true, as you know well, that a most successful—as the term goes—doctor may practise with a clinical slovenliness that makes it impossible for that kind old friend, Dame Nature, to cover his mistakes.

ON THE EDUCATIONAL VALUE OF A MEDICAL SOCIETY, IN AEQUANIMITAS, 342.

184. Mistakes in practicing medicine are not surprising.

It is astonishing with how little outside aid a large practice may be conducted, but it is not astonishing that in it cruel and unpardonable mistakes are made.

ON THE EDUCATIONAL VALUE OF THE MEDICAL SOCIETY. BOSTON MED SURG J
1903;147:275-9.

185. Do not promise cures.

We work by wit and not by witchcraft, and while these patients have our tenderest care, and we must do what is best for the relief of their sufferings, we should not bring the art of medicine into disrepute by quacklike promises to heal.

CUSHING H. THE LIFE OF WILLIAM OSLER, VOL. 2, 179.

186. Medicine is a jealous mistress.

Live a simple and a temperate life, that you may give all your powers to your profession. Medicine is a jealous mistress; she will be satisfied with no less.

THAYER WS. OSLER THE TEACHER, IN OSLER AND OTHER PAPERS, 4.

187. Professional work narrows the mind.

Professional work of any sort tends to narrow the mind, to limit the point of view and to put a hall-mark on a man of a most unmistakable kind.

THE MASTER-WORD IN MEDICINE, IN AEQUANIMITAS, 365.

188. The practitioner also needs culture.

One cannot practise medicine alone and practise it early and late, as so many of us have to do, and hope to escape the malign influences of a routine life. The incessant concentration of thought upon one subject, however interesting, tethers a man's mind in a narrow field. The practitioner needs culture as well as learning.

CHAUVINISM IN MEDICINE, IN AEQUANIMITAS, 285.

189. Culture counts in medicine.

In no profession does culture count for so much as in medicine, and no man needs it more than the general practitioner.

CHAUVINISM IN MEDICINE, IN AEQUANIMITAS, 285.

190. Warm your hands on the fire of life.

Amid the racket and hurly-burly [of practice] few of us have the chance to warm both hands at the fire of life.

BEAN WB. SIR WILLIAM OSLER: APHORISMS, 85.

191. Physicians must think.

The peril is that should he cease to think for himself he becomes a mere automaton, doing a penny-in-the-slot business which places him on a level with the chemist's clerk who can hand out specifics for every ill, from the "pip" [any unspecified human ailment] to the pox.

CHAUVINISM IN MEDICINE, IN AEQUANIMITAS, 283-4.

192. Practicing a penny-in-a-slot type of medicine is easy.

It is so much easier to do a penny-in-the-slot sort of practice, in which each symptom is at once met by its appropriate drug than to make a careful examination and really to study the case systematically.

THE IMPORTANCE OF POST-GRADUATE STUDY. LANCET 1900;2:73-5.

193. There are two sorts of doctors.

There are only two sorts of doctors; those who practise with their brains, and those who practise with their tongues.

TEACHING AND THINKING, IN AEQUANIMITAS, 124.

194. Many will need a strong leaven to practise.

Many of you will need a strong leaven to raise you above the dough in which it will be your lot to labour. Uncongenial surroundings, an ever-present dissonance between the aspirations within and the actualities without, the oppressive discords of human society, the bitter tragedies of life, the *lacrymae rerum* [inherent sadness], beside the hidden springs of which we sit in sad despair—all these tend to foster in some natures a cynicism quite foreign to our vocation, and to which this inner education offers the best antidote.

THE MASTER-WORD IN MEDICINE, IN AEQUANIMITAS, 367.

195. Institutional work can become routine.

Institutional life is very apt to get a person into a groove, which gets deeper and deeper until he cannot see over the edge of it.

COMMENCEMENT ADDRESS TO THE NURSES OF THE JOHNS HOPKINS TRAINING SCHOOL, MAY 7, 1913. JOHNS HOPKINS HOSP NURSES ALUM MAG 1913;12:72-81.

196. Take pride in caring for the poor.

In nothing should the citizens of a town take greater pride than in a well established, comfortable *Hôtel Dieu*—God's Hostelry—in which his poor are healed.

ON THE INFLUENCE OF A HOSPITAL UPON THE MEDICAL PROFESSION OF A COMMUNITY. ALBANY MED ANN 1901;22:1-11.

Financial and Material Interests of Practice

197. Deal with patients without considering financial return.

You have of course entered the Profession of Medicine with a view of obtaining a livelihood; but in dealing with your patients let this always be a secondary consideration.

VALEDICTORY ADDRESS TO THE GRADUATES IN MEDICINE AND SURGERY, MCGILL UNIVERSITY. CAN MED SURG J 1874-75;3:433-42.

198. The early intellectual rewards of medical practice will later bring financial return.

He [the physician at age 45] will probably have precious little capital in the bank, but a very large accumulation of interest-bearing funds in his brain-pan.

INTERNAL MEDICINE AS A VOCATION, IN AEQUANIMITAS, 141.

199. Medicine is a calling, not a business.

You are in this profession as a calling, not as a business; as a calling which exacts from you at every turn self-sacrifice, devotion, love and tenderness to your fellow-men. Once you get down to a purely business level, your influence is gone and the true light of your life is dimmed. You must work in the missionary spirit, with a breadth of charity that raises you far above the petty jealousies of life.

THE RESERVES OF LIFE. ST. MARY'S HOSP GAZ 1907;13:95-8.

200. Beware of a large and successful practice.

I would warn you against the trials of the day soon to come to some of you—the day of large and successful practice. Engrossed late and soon in professional cares, getting and spending, you may so lay waste your powers that you may find, too late, with hearts given away, that there is no place in your habit-stricken souls for those gentler influences which make life worth living.

AEQUANIMITAS, IN AEQUANIMITAS, 7

201. Prosperity can ruin.

Many good men are ruined by success in practice, and need to pray the prayer of the Litany against the evils of prosperity.

ON THE EDUCATIONAL VALUE OF THE MEDICAL SOCIETY, IN AEQUANIMITAS, 342.

202. *Some doctors become prosperous.*

Beyond a modest competency the sensible doctor does not aspire, but in the profession of every State there is a third group, composed of a few men who, dry-nursed by us, sometimes by the public, have become prosperous, perhaps wealthy. Freely they have received, freely they should give.

THE FUNCTIONS OF A STATE FACULTY. MARYLAND MED J 1897;37:73-77.

203. *Success is dangerous.*

The danger in such a man's life comes with prosperity. He is safe in the hard-working day, when he is climbing the hill, but once success is reached, with it come the temptations to which many succumb.

THE STUDENT LIFE, IN AEQUANIMITAS, 416-7.

204. *The medical profession must not value money above medicine.*

Fortunately the medical profession can never be wholly given over to commercialism, and perhaps this work of which we do so much, and for which we get so little—often not even thanks—is the best leaven against its corroding influence.

ON THE INFLUENCE OF A HOSPITAL UPON THE MEDICAL PROFESSION OF A COMMUNITY.

ALBANY MED ANN 1901;22:1-11.

205. *Consider the head, heart, and pocket in the professions.*

To combine in due measure the altruistic, the scientific and the business side of our work is not an easy task. In the three great professions, the lawyer has to consider only his head and pocket, the parson the head and the heart, while with us the head, heart, and pocket are all engaged.

REMARKS ON ORGANIZATION IN THE PROFESSION. BRIT MED J 1911;1:237-9.

206. *The physician's work is not, and must not, always be financially rewarding.*

The labourer is worthy of his hire, and the man in every trade and in many callings gets the cash equivalent for the daily round, but with us this can never be so. In every department of the [medical] profession the amount of unremunerative work is, and ever must be, enormous. . . . and the "good debts" of practice, as I prefer to call them . . . amount to a generous sum by the end of each year.

REMARKS ON ORGANIZATION IN THE PROFESSION. BRIT MED J 1911;1:237-9.

207. *Intellectual and moral standards protect against avarice.*

In the enormous development of material interests there is danger lest we miss altogether the secret of a nation's life, the true test of which is to be found in its intellectual and moral standards. There is no more potent antidote to the corroding influence of mammon than the presence in a community of a body of men devoted to science, living for investigation and caring nothing for the lust of the eyes and the pride of life.

TEACHER AND STUDENT, IN AEQUANIMITAS, 28.

208. *Beware of men calling you "Doc."*

Beware of the men that call you "Doc." They rarely pay their bills.

PRATT JH. A YEAR WITH OSLER, XIV

3

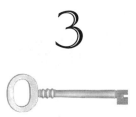

The Medical Profession

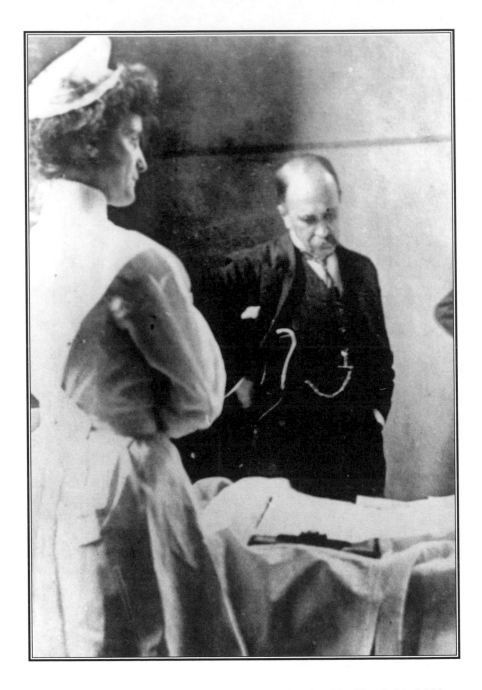

William Osler and nurse viewing the chart at Johns Hopkins Hospital in 1903.
(Courtesy of the Alan Mason Chesney Medical Archives
of the Johns Hopkins Medical Institutions.)

The Medical Profession

The Medical Profession

209. Medicine is an honored profession.

I would rather tell you of a profession honoured above all others; one which, while calling forth the highest powers of the mind, brings you into such warm personal contact with your fellow-men that the heart and sympathies of the coldest nature must needs be enlarged thereby.

INTRODUCTORY ADDRESS AT THE OPENING OF THE FORTY-FIFTH SESSION OF THE MEDICAL FACULTY, McGILL COLLEGE. CAN MED SURG J 1877-78;6:193-210.

210. Medicine is a noble heritage.

You enter a noble heritage, made so by no efforts of your own, but by the generations of men who have unselfishly sought to do the best they could for suffering mankind. Much has been done, much remains to do;

a way has been opened, and to the possibilities in the scientific development of medicine there seems to be no limit.

THE MASTER-WORD IN MEDICINE, IN AEQUANIMITAS, 370.

211. Fulfill the high mission of our noble calling.

In the student spirit you can best fulfil the high mission of our noble calling—in his *humility*, conscious of weakness, while seeking strength; in his *confidence*, knowing the power while recognizing the limitations of his art; in his *pride* in the glorious heritage from which the greatest gifts to man have been derived; and in his sure and certain hope that the future holds for us richer blessings than the past.

THE STUDENT LIFE, IN AEQUANIMITAS, 423.

212. Medical services are a sacred duty, done quietly.

Yours is a higher and more sacred duty. Think not to light a light before men that they may see your good works; contrariwise, you belong to the great army of quiet workers, physicians and priests, sisters and nurses, all over the world, the members of which strive not neither do they cry, nor are their voices heard in the streets, but to them is given the ministry of consolation in sorrow, need, and sickness.

THE MASTER-WORD IN MEDICINE, IN AEQUANIMITAS, 370.

213. Work and interest are keys to success.

The medical profession is one in which every man can make a success,...if he will work hard, study hard, and take an interest in his patients.

DR. OSLER TO STUDENTS. OKLAHOMA MED J 1900;8:53.

214. *The public has the right to expect a competent doctor.*

In a well-arranged community a citizen should feel that he can at any time command the services of a man who has received a fair training in the science and art of medicine, into whose hands he may commit with safety the lives of those near and dear to him.

THE GROWTH OF A PROFESSION. CAN MED SURG J 1885-86;14:129-55.

215. *Medicine has made major advances and has a great future.*

Never has the outlook for the profession been brighter. Everywhere the physician is better trained and better equipped than he was twenty-five years ago. Disease is understood more thoroughly, studied more carefully and treated more skilfully. The average sum of human suffering has been reduced in a way to make the angels rejoice. Diseases familiar to our fathers and grandfathers have disappeared, the death rate from others is falling to the vanishing point, and public health measures have lessened the sorrows and brightened the lives of millions. The vagaries and whims, lay and medical, may neither have diminished in number nor lessened in their capacity to distress the faint-hearted who do not appreciate that to the end of time people must imagine vain things, but they are dwarfed by comparison with the colossal advance of the past fifty years.

CHAUVINISM IN MEDICINE, IN AEQUANIMITAS, 269.

216. *Medicine is almost free of error and prejudice.*

Free, cosmopolitan, no longer hampered by the dogmas of schools, we may feel a just pride in a profession almost totally emancipated from the bondage of error and prejudice. Distinctions of race, nationality, colour, and creed are unknown within the portals of the temple of Aesculapius [Greek god of healing and patron deity of physicians]. Dare we dream that this harmony and cohesion so rapidly developing in medicine, obliterating the strongest lines of division, knowing no tie of loyalty, but loyalty to truth—dare we hope, I say, that in the wider range of human affairs a similar solidarity may ultimately be reached?

BRITISH MEDICINE IN GREATER BRITAIN, IN AEQUANIMITAS, 188.

217. Be aware of your own failings and avoid divisiveness.

The wrangling and unseemly disputes which have too often disgraced our profession arise, in a great majority of cases, on the one hand, from this morbid sensitiveness to the confession of error, and, on the other, from a lack of brotherly consideration, and a convenient forgetfulness of our own failings.

TEACHER AND STUDENT, IN AEQUANIMITAS, 39.

218. The calling of the physician is universal.

By his commission the physician is sent to the sick, and knowing in his calling neither Jew nor Gentile, bond or free, perhaps he alone rises superior to those differences which separate and make us dwell apart, too often oblivious to the common hopes and common frailties which should bind us together as a race. In his professional relations, though divided by national lines, there remains the feeling that he belongs to a Guild which owes no local allegiance, which has neither king nor country, but whose work is in the world. The Aesculapian temple has given place to the hospital, and the priestly character of the physician has vanished with the ages; still there is left with us a strong feeling of brotherhood, a sense of unity, which the limitations of language, race, and country have not been able to efface.

RUDOLPH VIRCHOW: THE MAN AND THE STUDENT. BOSTON MED SURG J
1891;125:425-7.

219. *Medicine is a world-wide guild of professionals of like mind and traditions.*

The profession in truth is a sort of guild or brotherhood, any member of which can take up his calling in any part of the world and find brethren whose language and methods and whose aims and ways are identical with his own.

CHAUVINISM IN MEDICINE, IN AEQUANIMITAS, 267.

220. *There is little room for chauvinism in medicine.*

With our History, Traditions, Achievements, and Hopes, there is little room for Chauvinism in medicine. The open mind, the free spirit of science, the ready acceptance of the best from any and every source, the attitude of rational receptiveness rather than of antagonism to new ideas, the liberal and friendly relationship between different nations and different sections of the same nation, the brotherly feeling which should characterize members of the oldest, most beneficent and universal guild that the race has evolved in its upward progress—these should neutralize the tendencies upon which I have so lightly touched.

CHAUVINISM IN MEDICINE, IN AEQUANIMITAS, 288.

221. *Nationalism can be a curse.*

Nationalism has been the great curse of humanity. In no other shape has the Demon of Ignorance assumed more hideous proportions; to no other obsession do we yield ourselves more readily. A vice of the blood, of the plasm rather, it runs riot in the race, and rages today as of yore in spite of the precepts of religion and the practice of democracy.

CHAUVINISM IN MEDICINE, IN AEQUANIMITAS, 271.

222. Each physician belongs to the profession, not himself.

No physician has a right to consider himself as belonging to himself; but all ought to regard themselves as belonging to the profession, inasmuch as each is a part of the profession; and care for the part naturally looks to care for the whole.

THE FUNCTIONS OF A STATE FACULTY. MARYLAND MED J 1897;37:73-7.

223. Medicine is the only world-wide profession.

Medicine is the only world-wide profession, following everywhere the same methods, actuated by the same ambitions, and pursuing the same ends. This homogeneity, its most characteristic feature, is not shared by the law, and not by the Church, certainly not in the same degree.

UNITY, PEACE AND CONCORD, IN AEQUANIMITAS, 429-30.

224. Medicine forms a remarkable world unit for hope.

Linked together by the strong bonds of community of interests, the profession of medicine forms a remarkable world-unit in the progressive evolution of which there is a fuller hope for humanity than in any other direction.

UNITY, PEACE AND CONCORD, IN AEQUANIMITAS, 432.

225. Medicine is universal.

Of no other profession is the word "universal" applicable in the same sense.... It is not the prevalence of disease or the existence everywhere of special groups of men to treat it that betokens this solidarity, but it is the identity throughout the civilized world of our ambitions, our methods and our work.

CHAUVINISM IN MEDICINE, IN AEQUANIMITAS, 267.

226. Medicine has no national boundaries.

The great Republic of Medicine knows and has known no national boundaries, and post-graduate study in other lands gives that broad mental outlook and that freedom from the trammels of local prejudice which have ever characterised the true physician.

THE IMPORTANCE OF POST-GRADUATE STUDY. LANCET 1900;2:73-5.

227. Harmony and unity of the medical profession is possible.

So vast, however, and composite has the profession become, that the physiological separation, in which dependent parts are fitly joined together, tends to become pathological, and while some parts suffer necrosis and degeneration, others, passing the normal limits, become disfiguring and dangerous outgrowths on the body medical. The dangers and evils which threaten harmony among the units, are internal, not external. And yet, in it more than in any other profession...is complete organic unity possible.

CHAUVINISM IN MEDICINE, IN AEQUANIMITAS, 269.

228. Practice in harmony with your medical colleagues.

Upon your relations to fellow-practitioners, allow me to offer you a few words of counsel. It is a fact well known to you all that the great opprobrium of our Profession, especially in the small towns, is the constant rivalry and distrust of one another displayed by its members. That men whose high calling ought to bind them closely together, and whose interest are so much in common, should thus disagree, is a matter deeply to be regretted; and, I would urge upon you, during your, let me hope, prosperous career, to do all that may lie in your power to remove this scandal from our midst.

VALEDICTORY ADDRESS TO THE GRADUATES IN MEDICINE AND SURGERY, MCGILL
UNIVERSITY. CAN MED SURG J 1874-75;3:433-42.

229. *Unity and friendship in the medical profession is important.*

The first, and in some respects the most important, function is that mentioned by the wise founders of your parent society—to lay a foundation for that unity and friendship which is essential to the dignity and usefulness of the profession. Unity and friendship! How we all long for them, but how difficult to attain! Strife seems rather to be the very life of the practitioner, whose warfare is incessant against disease and against ignorance and prejudice, and, sad to have to admit, he too often lets his angry passions rise against his professional brother. The quarrels of doctors make a pretty chapter in the history of medicine.

On the Educational Value of the Medical Society, in Aequanimitas, 335-6.

230. *The good feeling and conditions of professional life are everywhere.*

One of the most gratifying features of our professional life is the good feeling which prevails between the various sections of the country.... One has only to visit different parts and mingle with the men to appreciate that everywhere good work is being done, everywhere an earnest desire to elevate the standard of education, and everywhere the same self-sacrificing devotion on the part of the general practitioner. Men will tell you that commercialism is rife, that the charlatan and the humbug were never so much in evidence, and that in our ethical standards there has been a steady declension. These are the Elijahs who are always ready to pour out their complaints, mourning that they are not better than their fathers. Few men have had more favourable opportunities than I have had to gauge the actual conditions in professional private life, in the schools, and in the medical societies, and...I am filled with thankfulness for the present and with hope for the future.

Unity, Peace and Concord, in Aequanimitas, 438-9.

231. *Have faith in the profession.*

I have had faith in the profession, the most unbounded confidence in it as one of the great factors in the progress of humanity; and one of the special satisfactions of my life has been that my brethren have in many practical ways shown faith in me, often much more than (as I know in my heart of hearts) I have deserved.

THE FAITH THAT HEALS. BRIT MED J 1910;1:1470-2.

232. *Do not listen to malcontents.*

Some will tell you that the profession is underrated, unhonoured, underpaid, its members social drudges—the very last profession they would recommend a young man to take up. Listen not to these croakers; there are such in every calling, and the secret of their discontent is not hard to discover. The evils which they deprecate and ascribe—it is difficult to say to whom—in themselves lie; evils, the seeds of which were sown when they were students; sown in hours of idleness, in inattention to studies, in consequent failure to grasp those principles of their science without which the practice of medicine does indeed become a drudgery, for it degenerates into a business.

MEDICINE AND NURSING. IN MATHEWS B (ED). ESSAYS ON VOCATION. LONDON: OXFORD UNIVERSITY PRESS, 1919:8.

233. *Uncertainty is the rule in medicine.*

Gentlemen, if you want a profession in which everything is certain you had better give up medicine.

MCCRAE T. THE INFLUENCE OF PATHOLOGY ON THE CLINICAL MEDICINE OF WILLIAM OSLER. IN ABBOTT ME (ED). SIR WILLIAM OSLER MEMORIAL NUMBER. BULLETIN NO. IX OF THE INTERNATIONAL ASSOCIATION OF MEDICAL MUSEUMS AND JOURNAL OF TECHNICAL METHODS. MONTREAL: PRIVATELY PRINTED, 1926:39.

234. Medicine is distinguished by its singular beneficence.

Not that we all live up to the highest ideals, far from it—we are only men. But we have ideals, which means much—and they are realizable, which means more…. Of course there are Gehazis [Biblical—Elisha's dishonest servant] among us who serve for shekels, whose ears hear only the lowing of the oxen and the jingling of the guineas, but these are exceptions. The rank and file labour earnestly for good, and self-sacrificing devotion animates our best work.

MEDICINE AND NURSING. IN MATHEWS B (ED). ESSAYS ON VOCATION. LONDON:
OXFORD UNIVERSITY PRESS, 1919:5.

235. Show enthusiasm for your chosen work.

Lukewarmness, bad enough at any time, is simply fatal at the beginning of a life-long career, when it usurps the place of that enthusiasm that should bend the man's whole nature to serve him willingly in the work he has chosen.

INTRODUCTORY ADDRESS AT THE OPENING OF THE FORTY-FIFTH SESSION OF THE
MEDICAL FACULTY, MCGILL COLLEGE. CAN MED SURG J 1877-78;6:193-210.

236. Interest in profession leads to success.

The very first step towards success in any occupation is to become interested in it… And there is nothing more certain than that you cannot study well if you are not interested in your profession.

THE MASTER-WORD IN MEDICINE, IN AEQUANIMITAS, 359.

Medical Societies

237. The medical society can prevent a stale mind.

We doctors do not "take stock" often enough, and are very apt to carry on our shelves stale, out-of-date goods. The society helps to keep a man "up to the times," and enables him to refurnish his mental shop with the latest wares. Rightly used, it may be a touchstone to which he can bring his experiences to the test and save him from falling into the rut of a few sequences. It keeps his mind open and receptive, and counteracts that tendency to premature senility which is apt to overtake a man who lives in a routine.

ON THE MEDICAL SOCIETY, IN AEQUANIMITAS, 337.

238. Medical societies promote harmony and good-fellowship.

By no means the smallest advantage [of medical societies] is the promotion of harmony and good-fellowship. Medical men, particularly in smaller places, live too much apart and do not see enough of each other. In large cities, we rub each other's angles down and carom off each other without feeling the shock very much, but it is an unfortunate circumstance that in many towns the friction, being on a small surface, hurts; and mutual misunderstandings arise to the destruction of all harmony.

THE GROWTH OF A PROFESSION. CAN MED SURG J 1885-86;14:129-55.

239. Be involved in professional associations.

You cannot afford to stand aloof from your professional colleagues in any place. Join their associations, mingle in their meetings, giving of the best of your talents, gathering here, scattering there; but everywhere showing that you are at all times faithful students, as willing to teach as to be taught.

THE ARMY SURGEON, IN AEQUANIMITAS, 110.

240. Discord, jealousy, and faction in medicine can be overcome.

Of the value to the local practitioner of a medical society and of a library we are all agreed. How common the experience to enter a cold cheerless room in which the fire in the grate has died down, not from lack of coal, not because the coal was not alight, but the bits, large and small, falling away from each other, have gradually become dark and cold. Break them with a poker, get them together, and what a change in a few minutes! There is light and heat and good cheer. What happens in the grate illustrates very often the condition of the profession in a town or county; single or in cliques the men have fallen apart, and, as in the dead or dying embers, there is neither light nor warmth; or the coals may be there alive and bright, but covered with the ashes of discord, jealousy, and faction.

REMARKS ON ORGANIZATION IN THE PROFESSION. BRIT MED J 1911;1:237-9.

241. Pity the hurried practitioner.

Of all men in the profession the forty-visit-a-day man is the most to be pitied. Not always an automaton, he may sometimes by economy of words and extraordinary energy do his work well, but too often he is the one above all others who needs the refreshment of mind and recreation that is to be had in a well-conducted society.

ON THE EDUCATION AND VALUE OF THE MEDICAL SOCIETY, IN AEQUANIMITAS, 342.

242. The medical society is a corrective to egoism.

No class of men need friction so much as physicians; no class gets less. The daily round of a busy practitioner tends to develop an egoism of a most intense kind, to which there is no antidote. The few set-backs are forgotten. The mistakes are often buried, and ten years of successful work tends to make a man touchy, dogmatic, intolerant of correction and abominably self-centered. To this mental attitude the medical society is the best corrective, and a man misses a good part of his education who does not get knocked about a bit by his colleagues in discussions and criticisms.

THE FUNCTIONS OF A STATE FACULTY. MARYLAND MED J 1897;37:73-7.

The Doctor

243. Family medicine has great rewards.

It cannot be denied that…there are fewer great prizes open to the medical man than to others from whom a long and special training is demanded. He is not raised to command his fellow-men; his name is not immortalized in history and song like those of the gallant veterans who wear her Majesty's uniform, and risk their lives for their country and their Queen; he does not sit among the judges of the land; the high places of brilliant statesmanship are not for him; while the world at large can reward him with little beyond a successful practice in which every dollar that he earns represents its equivalent in hard continuous work. But while the soldier and the statesman win honour and fame, the family physician will draw to himself the love and gratitude of manifold hearts; he will have no enemies, martial or political; and his labours if directed by a wise and prudent skill, will be for the welfare and benefit of all.

INTRODUCTORY ADDRESS AT THE OPENING OF THE FORTY-FIFTH SESSION OF THE
MEDICAL FACULTY, McGILL COLLEGE. CAN MED SURG J 1877-78;6:193-210.

244. The ideals of medicine are expressed through the work of the general practitioner.

I have an enduring faith in the men who do the routine work of our profession. Hard though the conditions may be, approached in the right spirit—the spirit which has animated us from the days of Hippocrates—the practice of medicine affords scope for the exercise of the best faculties of the mind and heart. That the yoke of the general practitioner is often galling cannot be denied, but he has not a monopoly of the worries and trials in the meeting and conquering of which he fights his life battle.

PREFACE, IN AEQUANIMITAS, VII.

245. The family doctor is on the front line of fighting.

The family doctor, the private in our great army, the essential factor in the battle, should be carefully nurtured by the schools and carefully guarded by the public. Humanly speaking, with him are the issues of life and death, since upon him falls the grievous responsibility in those terrible emergencies which bring darkness and despair to so many households.

ON THE EDUCATIONAL VALUE OF THE MEDICAL SOCIETY, IN AEQUANIMITAS, 331.

246. The general practitioner has noble character.

The cultivated general practitioner. May this be the destiny of a large majority of you!...You cannot reach any better position in a community; the family doctor is the man behind the gun, who does our effective work. That his life is hard and exacting; that he is underpaid and overworked; that he has but little time for study and less for recreation—these are the blows that may give finer temper to his steel, and bring out the nobler elements in his character.

THE STUDENT LIFE, IN AEQUANIMITAS, 410-1.

247. A well-trained doctor is a valuable asset.

A well-trained, sensible doctor is one of the most valuable assets of a community, worth to-day, as in Homer's time, many another man. To make him efficient is our highest ambition as teachers, to save him from evil should be our constant care as a guild.

CHAUVINISM IN MEDICINE, IN AEQUANIMITAS, 281.

248. Maintaining mental freshness requires vigilance.

To maintain mental freshness and plasticity requires incessant vigilance; too often, like the dial's hand, it steals from its figure with no pace perceived except by one's friends, and they never refer to it. A deep and an enduring interest in the manifold problems of medicine and a human interest in the affairs of our brotherhood—if these do not suffice nothing will.

THE IMPORTANCE OF POST-GRADUATE STUDY. LANCET 1900;2:73-5.

249. The physician has three great foes.

The physician...has three great foes—ignorance, which is sin; apathy, which is the world; and vice, which is the devil.... Teaching the simple and suffering the fools gladly, we must fight the wilful ignorance of the one and the helpless ignorance of the other, not with the sword of righteous indignation, but with the skilful weapon of the tongue.

UNITY, PEACE AND CONCORD, IN AEQUANIMITAS, 435-6.

250. We are easily misled by our experience.

And not only are the reactions [of patients] themselves variable, but we, the doctors, are so fallible, ever beset with the common and fatal facility of reaching conclusions from superficial observations, and constantly misled by the ease with which our minds fall into the ruts of one or two experiences.

TEACHER AND STUDENT, IN AEQUANIMITAS, 35-6.

251. To be misunderstood often provokes indignation.

When one has done his best or when a mistake has arisen through lack of special knowledge, but more particularly when, as so often happens, our heart's best sympathies have been engaged, to be misunderstood by the patient and his friends, to have evil motives imputed and to be maligned, is too much for human endurance, and justifies a righteous indignation.

CHAUVINISM IN MEDICINE, IN AEQUANIMITAS, 287.

252. Doctors do not take criticism well.

More perhaps than any other professional man, the doctor has a curious—shall I say morbid?—sensitiveness to (what he regards) personal error. In a way this is right; but it is too often accompanied by a *cocksureness* of opinion which, if encouraged, leads him to so lively a conceit that the mere suggestion of mistake under any circumstances is regarded as a reflection on his honour, a reflection equally resented whether of lay or of professional origin.

TEACHER AND STUDENT, IN AEQUANIMITAS, 38.

253. Physicians dislike authority.

Physicians, as a rule, have less appreciation of the value of organization than the members of other professions.

THE FUNCTIONS OF A STATE FACULTY. MARYLAND MED J 1897;37:73-7.

254. Don't treat yourself.

A physician who treats himself has a fool for a patient.

BEAN WB. SIR WILLIAM OSLER: APHORISMS, 53.

255. Take care of yourself.

In no relationship is the physician more often derelict than in his duty to himself.

DR. JOHNSTON AS A PHYSICIAN. WASHINGTON MED ANN 1902;1:158-61.

256. Halitosis is common in the population, including physicians.

The practitioner is frequently consulted for foul breath, and is daily made aware of its wide-spread prevalence. Too often he is himself the subject of the condition, to the disgust of his patients, with whom he has to come into such close contact.

THE PRINCIPLES AND PRACTICE OF MEDICINE, 439.

257. Do not sacrifice mental independence.

In no single relation of life does the general practitioner show a more illiberal spirit than in the treatment of himself. I do not refer so much to careless habits of living, to lack of routine in work, or to failure to pay due attention to the business side of the profession—sins which so easily beset him—but I would speak of his failure to realize *first,* the need of a lifelong progressive personal training, and *secondly,* the danger lest in the stress of practice he sacrifice that most precious of all possessions, his mental independence.

CHAUVINISM IN MEDICINE, IN AEQUANIMITAS, 281.

258. Slow the engines of life.

Much depends on the patient himself—on the life he has led—the life he is willing to lead. The ordinary high-pressure business or professional man may find relief, or even cure, in the simple process of slowing the engines, reducing the speed from the 25 knots an hour of a *Lusitania* to the 10 knots of a "black Bilbao tramp [from "L'envoi" by Rudyard Kipling (1865-1936)]." The difficulty is to induce a man of this type to lessen "the race, an' rack, an' strain".... We doctors are notorious sinners in this respect, but it is so hard to lessen work when in full swing, so much harder than to give up altogether, and how few of us at 50 or 55 are able to do this!

LUMLEIAN LECTURES ON ANGINA PECTORIS. LANCET 1910;1:973-7.

259. Respect your colleagues.

Respect your colleagues. Know that there is no more high-minded body of men than the medical profession.

THAYER, WS. OSLER THE TEACHER, IN OSLER AND OTHER PAPERS, 2.

260. A surgeon's career is shorter than a physician's career.

The surgeon grows more rapidly than the physician, matures earlier, but rarely lasts so long.

ON THE INFLUENCE OF A HOSPITAL UPON THE MEDICAL PROFESSION OF A COMMUNITY.

ALBANY MED ANN 1901;22:1-11.

The Specialists

261. There are no specialties in medicine.

There are, in truth, no specialties in medicine, since to know fully many of the most important diseases a man must be familiar with their manifestations in many organs.

THE ARMY SURGEON, IN AEQUANIMITAS, 104.

262. The wise counsel of the specialist is comforting.

How comforting to the general practitioner is the wise counsel of the specialist. We take him a case that has puzzled and annoyed us, the diagnosis of which is uncertain, and we consult in vain the unwritten records of our experience and the printed records of our books. He labels it in a few minutes as a coleopterist [insect specialist] would a beetle, and we feel grateful for the accuracy of his information and happy in the possession of the label.

REMARKS ON SPECIALISM. BOSTON MED SURG J 1892;126:457-9.

263. Assurance and counseling are an important function of the consultant.

In others the chief value of the consultation has been in a reasonable talk with the patient about his condition, with assurance that there was nothing serious, and general advice as to mode of life and diet. Coleridge [English poet, 1772-1834] somewhere remarks that when a man is vaguely ill the talk of a doctor about the nature of his malady tones him down and consoles. It is very true, and to tone down and console are important functions of professional advisers.

CAMAC CNB. COUNSELS AND IDEALS. BOSTON: HOUGHTON MIFFLIN, 1929:213.

264. Specialization has expanded our knowledge.

The restriction of the energies of trained students to narrow fields in science, while not without its faults, has been the most important single factor in the remarkable expansion of our knowledge. Against the disadvantages in a loss of breadth and harmony there is the compensatory benefit of a greater accuracy in the application of knowledge in specialism, as is well illustrated in the cultivation of special branches of practice.

MEDICINE IN THE NINETEENTH CENTURY, IN AEQUANIMITAS, 224.

265. The public desires a medical specialist.

It is almost unnecessary to remark that the public, in which we live and move, has not been slow to recognize the advantage of a division of labor in the field of medicine. The desire for expert knowledge is, however, now so general that there is a grave danger lest the family doctor should become, in some places, a relic of the past.

REMARKS ON SPECIALISM. BOSTON MED SURG J 1892;126:457-9.

266. Work together for the benefit of the community.

Members of a corporate body, successful life will depend upon the permeation by harmonics which correlate and control the functions. Isolation means organic inadequacy—each must work in sympathy and in union with the other and all for the benefit of the community—all toward what Bacon [English philosopher and essayist, 1561-1626] calls the lawful goal of the sciences, that human life be endowed with new discoveries and power.

SPECIALISM IN THE GENERAL HOSPITAL. JOHNS HOPKINS HOSP BULL 1913;24:167-71.

267. There are disadvantages of specialization.

Specialism is not, however, without many disadvantages. A radical error at the onset is the failure to recognize that the results of specialized observation are at best only partial truths, which require to be correlated with facts obtained by wider study. The various organs, the diseases of which are subdivided for treatment, are not isolated, but complex parts of a complex whole, and every day's experience brings home the truth of the saying, "When one member suffers all the members suffer with it."

REMARKS ON SPECIALISM. BOSTON MED SURG J 1892;126:457-9.

268. The weak specialist is dangerous.

The dangers do not come to the strong man in a speciality, but to the weak brother who seeks it in an easier field in which specious garrulity and mechanical dexterity may take the place of solid knowledge. All goes well when the man is larger than his speciality and controls it, but when the speciality runs away with the man there is disaster, and a topsy-turvy condition, which in every branch, has done incalculable injury.

THE STUDENT LIFE, IN AEQUANIMITAS, 419.

269. Early specialization is dangerous.

No more dangerous members of our profession exist than those born into it, so to speak, as specialists. Without any broad foundation in physiology or pathology, and ignorant of the great processes of disease no amount of technical skill can hide from the keen eyes of colleagues defects which too often require the arts of the charlatan to screen from the public.

REMARKS ON SPECIALISM. BOSTON MED SURG J 1892;126:457-9.

270. Concentrating narrows the mind.

The incessant concentration of thought upon one subject, however interesting, tethers a man's mind in a narrow field.

CHAUVINISM IN MEDICINE, IN AEQUANIMITAS, 285.

271. A specialist tends to be narrow in spirit.

In the cultivation of a specialty as an *art* there is a tendency to develop a narrow and pedantic spirit; and the man who, year in and year out examines eyes, palpates ovaries, or tunnels urethrae, without regard to the wider influences upon which his art rests, is apt, insensibly perhaps, but none the less surely, to acquire the attitude of mind of the old Scotch shoemaker, who, in response to Dominie's suggestions about the weightier matters of life, asked, "D'ye ken leather?" [from *Guy Mannering* by Sir Walter Scott (1771-1832)]

REMARKS ON SPECIALISM. BOSTON MED SURG J 1892;126:457-9.

272. Experience can be skewed.

Seeing the more severe cases, the experience of the consultant is apt to be misleading.

LUMLEIAN LECTURES ON ANGINA PECTORIS. LANCET 1910;1:973-7.

273. Consultants may suffer intellectual idleness.

We all have our therapeutic ruts, and we all know consultants from whom patients find it very difficult to escape without their favourite prescription, no matter what the malady may be. Men of this stamp gain a certain measure of experience, and if of a practical turn of mind may become experts in mechanical procedures, but to experience in the true sense of the word they never attain. In reality they suffer from the all-prevailing vice of intellectual idleness.

THE IMPORTANCE OF POST-GRADUATE STUDY. LANCET 1900;2:73-5.

274. Internal medicine is hard to delineate.

I wish there were another term to designate the wide field of medical practice which remains after the separation of surgery, midwifery, and gynaecology. Not itself a specialty, (though it embraces at least half a dozen), its cultivators cannot be called specialists, but bear without reproach the good old name physician, in contradistinction to general practitioners, surgeons, obstetricians and gynaecologists.... At the outset I would like to emphasize the fact that the student of internal medicine cannot be a specialist.

INTERNAL MEDICINE AS A VOCATION, IN AEQUANIMITAS, 133.

275. The chief function of a consultant is to do a rectal exam.

The chief function of the consultant is to make a rectal examination that you have omitted.

BEAN WB. SIR WILLIAM OSLER: APHORISMS, 104.

The Nurse

276. There is no higher mission in life than nursing.

There is no higher mission in this life than nursing God's poor. In so doing a woman may not reach the ideals of her soul; she may fall far short of the ideals of her head, but she will go far to satiate those longings of the heart from which no woman can escape.

NURSE AND PATIENT, IN AEQUANIMITAS, 158.

277. The trained nurse is one of the great blessings of humanity.

The trained nurse has become one of the great blessings of humanity, taking a place beside the physician and the priest, and not inferior to either in her mission.... Time out of mind she has made one of a trinity.... Kindly heads have always been ready to devise means for allaying suffering; tender hearts, surcharged with the miseries of this "battered caravanserai" [an oriental inn], have ever been ready to speak to the sufferer of a way of peace, and loving hands have ever ministered to those in sorrow, need and sickness.

NURSE AND PATIENT, IN AEQUANIMITAS, 156.

278. Caring is an old tradition; nursing as a profession is new.

Nursing as an art to be cultivated, as a profession to be followed, is modern; nursing as a practice originated in the dim past, when some mother among the cave-dwellers cooled the forehead of her sick child with water from the brook, or first yielded to the prompting to leave a well-covered bone and a handful of meal by the side of a wounded man left in the hurried flight before an enemy.

NURSE AND PATIENT, IN AEQUANIMITAS, 156-7.

279. Gentleness is the nurse's birthright.

Gentleness is your birthright as a nurse. It is expressed by words, by hand or in motion.

COMMENCEMENT ADDRESS TO THE NURSES OF THE JOHNS HOPKINS TRAINING SCHOOL, MAY 7, 1913. JOHNS HOPKINS HOSP NURSES ALUM MAG 1913;12:72-81.

280. Nurses have seven virtues.

There are seven [virtues], the mystic seven, your lamps to lighten your work and they are tact, tidiness, taciturnity, sympathy, gentleness, cheerfulness, all linked together by charity.

COMMENCEMENT ADDRESS TO THE NURSES OF THE JOHNS HOPKINS TRAINING SCHOOL, MAY 7, 1913. JOHNS HOPKINS HOSP NURSES ALUM MAG 1913;12:72-81.

281. The nurse sees the undraped and fully revealed person.

No other people in the world see men and women as the private nurse does. She sees them, as I once said before, in mufti [out of uniform], with all of their mental and moral, and many of their bodily clothes taken off. For a student of human nature there is no other such profession.

COMMENCEMENT ADDRESS TO THE NURSES OF THE JOHNS HOPKINS TRAINING SCHOOL, MAY 7, 1913. JOHNS HOPKINS HOSP NURSES ALUM MAG 1913;12:72-81.

282. Nurses should be nonjudgmental.

Gently to scan your brother man, still more gently your sister woman, to judge no one harshly, to live as closely as possible to the counsels of the Sermon on the Mount, may enable you to live in the true spirit of nursing. These riches shall not fade away in life, nor any death decrease.

COMMENCEMENT ADDRESS TO THE NURSES OF THE JOHNS HOPKINS TRAINING SCHOOL, MAY 7, 1913. JOHNS HOPKINS HOSP NURSES ALUM MAG 1913;12:72-81.

283. Be blind to the faults of nurses.

The trained nurse as a factor in life may be regarded from many points of view—philanthropic, social, personal, professional and domestic. To her virtues we have been exceedingly kind—tongues have dropped manna in their description. To her faults—well let us be blind.

NURSE AND PATIENT, IN AEQUANIMITAS, 149.

284. Nurses should marry.

Marriage is the natural end of the trained nurse. So truly as a young man married is a young man marred, is a woman unmarried, in a certain sense, a woman undone.

NURSE AND PATIENT, IN AEQUANIMITAS, 155.

285. *The doctor and the nurse have evolved as useful partners.*

In the gradual division of labour, by which civilization has emerged from barbarism, the doctor and the nurse have been evolved, as useful accessories in the incessant warfare in which man is engaged.

DOCTOR AND NURSE, IN AEQUANIMITAS, 17.

4

Diagnosis

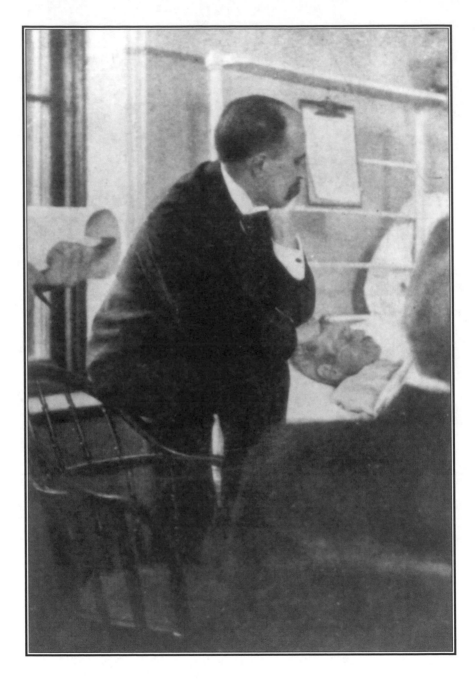

William Osler contemplating at the bedside at Johns Hopkins Hospital in 1903.
(Courtesy of the Alan Mason Chesney Medical Archives
of the Johns Hopkins Medical Institutions.)

Diagnosis

Examination

286. *Methodical examination leads to safe inductions.*

It is only by the methodical examination of every system and organ that we get those comprehensive facts from which we can draw reasonably safe inductions.

UNPUBLISHED DRAFT OF AN ADDRESS TO MEDICAL STUDENTS AT THE UNIVERSITY OF PENNSYLVANIA, 1885. PUBLISHED PRIVATELY BY THE OSLER LIBRARY, MCGILL UNIVERSITY, MONTREAL, 2006.

287. Listen to the patient.

Listen to the patient, he is telling you the diagnosis.

SOURCE UNCERTAIN. FREQUENTLY ATTRIBUTED TO WILLIAM OSLER AND INSCRIBED ON A MEDAL IN HIS HONOR BY DR. MASAKAZU ABE, JIKEI MEDICAL COLLEGE, JAPAN, 1968.

288. Know the normal before examining for the abnormal.

To be able to recognize abnormal states, you must bring a full knowledge of the normal situation of the organs, their physical signs, and the characters and composition of the excretions. Without these standards of comparison, you cannot make the first step in the examination of your patient.

UNPUBLISHED DRAFT OF AN ADDRESS TO MEDICAL STUDENTS AT THE UNIVERSITY OF PENNSYLVANIA, 1885. PUBLISHED PRIVATELY BY THE OSLER LIBRARY, MCGILL UNIVERSITY, MONTREAL, 2006.

289. Collect all the facts first.

But the sick man is before you. How shall you proceed in your examination? He represents a complicated experience or problem and the first thing to do is to collect all the facts of the case.

UNPUBLISHED DRAFT OF AN ADDRESS TO MEDICAL STUDENTS AT THE UNIVERSITY OF PENNSYLVANIA, 1885. PUBLISHED PRIVATELY BY THE OSLER LIBRARY, MCGILL UNIVERSITY, MONTREAL, 2006.

290. The art of medicine is in observation.

The whole art of medicine is in observation...but to educate the eye to see, the ear to hear and the finger to feel takes time, and to make a beginning, to start a man on the right path, is all that we can do.

On the Need of a Radical Reform in Our Methods of Teaching Senior Students. Med News [New York] 1903;82:49-53.

291. The difficult art of observation is hard to acquire.

There is no more difficult art to acquire than the art of observation, and for some men it is quite as difficult to record an observation in brief and plain language.

On the Educational Value of the Medical Society, in Aequanimitas, 340.

292. See first.

See, and then reason and compare and control. But see first. No two eyes see the same thing. No two mirrors give forth the same reflexion.

Thayer WS. Osler the Teacher, in Osler and Other Papers, 1.

293. See straight and think clearly.

Observation *plus* thinking has given us the vast stores of knowledge we now possess of the structure of the bodies of living creatures in health and disease. There have been two inherent difficulties—to get men to see straight and to get men to think clearly; but in spite of the frailty of the instrument, the method has been one of the most powerful ever placed in the hands of man.

The Pathological Institute of a General Hospital. Glasgow Med J 1911;76:321-33.

294. *Observe and profit.*

But it is by your own eyes, and your ears and your own mind and (I may add) your own heart that you must observe and learn and profit.

BEAN WB. SIR WILLIAM OSLER: APHORISMS, 121.

295. *Routine and system facilitate work.*

Routine and system when once made a habit, facilitate work, and the busier you are the more time you will have to make observations after examining a patient.

THE STUDENT LIFE, IN AEQUANIMITAS, 412.

296. *Our experience can be misleading.*

We, the doctors, are so fallible, ever beset with the common fatal facility of reaching conclusions from superficial observations, and constantly misled by the ease with which our minds fall into the ruts of one or two experiences.

TEACHER AND STUDENT, IN AEQUANIMITAS, 35-6.

297. *Memory distorts the facts.*

Memory plays strange pranks with facts. The rocks and fissures and gullies of the mountain-side melt quickly into the smooth, blue outlines of the distant panorama. Viewed through the perspective of memory, an unrecorded observation, the vital details long since lost, easily changes its countenance and sinks obediently into the frame fashioned by the fancy of the moment.

THAYER WS. OSLER THE TEACHER, IN OSLER AND OTHER PAPERS, 1.

298. Ask no leading questions.

In taking histories follow each line of thought; ask no leading questions; never suggest. Give the patient's own words in the complaint.

BEAN WB. SIR WILLIAM OSLER: APHORISMS, 41.

299. The occupation may point to the diagnosis.

It is always valuable to note the occupation of a patient. It may point to the diagnosis of the disease. The fact that a man with anomalous symptoms and a cutaneous eruption is a wool sorter may give the diagnosis of anthrax. Glanders is associated with workers in stables.... When a man with extreme pallor says he is a painter, this fact at once points to lead poisoning as the cause. The same with tailors as there is lead in the thread they use.

PRATT JH. A YEAR WITH OSLER, 1-2.

300. Abdominal pain may be due to a morphine habit.

Severe pains in the abdomen and recurring attacks of colic without definite cause lead one to suspect the patient has the morphine habit.

PRATT JH. A YEAR WITH OSLER, 38.

301. There are four points to a medical student's compass.

The four points of a medical student's compass are: Inspection, Palpation, Percussion, and Auscultation.

BEAN WB. SIR WILLIAM OSLER: APHORISMS, 103.

302. Pay attention to your bedside manner.

Remember, however, that every patient upon whom you wait will examine you critically and form an estimate of you by the way in which you conduct yourself at the bedside. Skill and nicety in manipulation, whether in the simple act of feeling the pulse, or in the performance of any minor operation will do more towards establishing confidence in you, than a string of Diplomas, or the reputation of extensive Hospital experience.

VALEDICTORY ADDRESS TO THE GRADUATES IN MEDICINE AND SURGERY, McGILL UNIVERSITY. CAN MED SURG J 1874-75;3:433-42.

303. Use your five senses.

Get the patient in a good light. Use your five senses. We miss more by not seeing than we do by not knowing. Always examine the back. Observe, record, tabulate, communicate.

ROBERTS SR. WILLIAM OSLER, CLINICIAN-TEACHER. IN ABBOTT ME (ED). SIR WILLIAM OSLER MEMORIAL NUMBER. BULLETIN NO. IX OF THE INTERNATIONAL ASSOCIATION OF MEDICAL MUSEUMS AND JOURNAL OF TECHNICAL METHODS. MONTREAL: PRIVATELY PRINTED, 1926:432.

304. Make a thorough inspection.

Make a thorough inspection. Never forget to look at the back of a patient. Always look at the feet. Looking at a woman's legs has often saved her life.

BEAN WB. SIR WILLIAM OSLER: APHORISMS, 104.

305. We are all deaf.

Half of us are blind, few of us feel, and we are all deaf.

BEAN WB. SIR WILLIAM OSLER: APHORISMS, 37.

306. Examine the throat and the rectum.

Failure to examine the throat is a glaring sin of omission, especially in children. One finger in the throat and one in the rectum makes a good diagnostician.

BEAN WB. SIR WILLIAM OSLER: APHORISMS, 104.

307. Tune up your auditory cells.

When listening to heart murmurs you must tune up your auditory hair cells and flatten out your Pacinian corpuscles.

BEAN WB. SIR WILLIAM OSLER: APHORISMS, 104.

308. A giant colon is all about wind.

On palpation of a giant colon: Where you expect water you find wind, no land anywhere.

BEAN WB. SIR WILLIAM OSLER: APHORISMS, 147.

Diagnosis

309. Put the patient before the disease.

There is a tendency among young men about hospitals to study the cases, not the patients, and in the interest they take in the disease lose sight of the individual. Strive against this.

UNPUBLISHED DRAFT OF AN ADDRESS TO MEDICAL STUDENTS AT THE UNIVERSITY OF PENNSYLVANIA, 1885. PUBLISHED PRIVATELY BY THE OSLER LIBRARY, McGILL UNIVERSITY, MONTREAL, 2006.

310. Diagnosis and treatment are your tasks.

Two thoughts should ever be in your minds: how can I best recognize and how can I best treat disease.

UNPUBLISHED DRAFT OF AN ADDRESS TO MEDICAL STUDENTS AT THE UNIVERSITY OF PENNSYLVANIA, 1885. PUBLISHED PRIVATELY BY THE OSLER LIBRARY, MCGILL UNIVERSITY, MONTREAL, 2006.

311. Each case is different.

One element must always be taken into account in prognosis and that is the personal equation of the patient. No two cases of the same disease are ever alike; the constitution of the person, his individuality, stamps each case with certain peculiarities.

UNPUBLISHED DRAFT OF AN ADDRESS TO MEDICAL STUDENTS AT THE UNIVERSITY OF PENNSYLVANIA, 1885. PUBLISHED PRIVATELY BY THE OSLER LIBRARY, MCGILL UNIVERSITY, MONTREAL, 2006.

312. Be satisfied with probabilities in diagnosis.

You will soon learn, however, in practice, to be satisfied with probabilities.

UNPUBLISHED DRAFT OF AN ADDRESS TO MEDICAL STUDENTS AT THE UNIVERSITY OF PENNSYLVANIA, 1885. PUBLISHED PRIVATELY BY THE OSLER LIBRARY, MCGILL UNIVERSITY, MONTREAL, 2006.

313. Overconfidence leads to a rude awakening.

Various degrees of probability we may attain to and do reach daily but in the busy round of teaching and practice we are apt to forget that positive certainty until we have a rude awakening and a useful lesson in the folly of over-confidence.

UNPUBLISHED DRAFT OF AN ADDRESS TO MEDICAL STUDENTS AT THE UNIVERSITY OF PENNSYLVANIA, 1885. PUBLISHED PRIVATELY BY THE OSLER LIBRARY, MCGILL UNIVERSITY, MONTREAL, 2006.

314. Keep an open mind or you will be dogmatic.

Come to the study of the diagnosis of disease with all the modesty at your command. Positiveness and dogmatism are inevitable associates of superficial knowledge in medicine.

UNPUBLISHED DRAFT OF AN ADDRESS TO MEDICAL STUDENTS AT THE UNIVERSITY OF PENNSYLVANIA, 1885. PUBLISHED PRIVATELY BY THE OSLER LIBRARY, MCGILL UNIVERSITY, MONTREAL, 2006.

315. These are our methods and our work.

To carefully observe the phenomena of life in all its phases, normal and perverted, to make perfect that most difficult of all arts, the art of observation, to call to aid the science of experimentation, to cultivate the reasoning faculty, so as to be able to know the true from the false—these are our methods. To prevent disease, to relieve suffering and to heal the sick—this is our work.

CHAUVINISM IN MEDICINE, IN AEQUANIMITAS, 267.

316. Diagnosis is our chief weapon.

In the fight which we have to wage incessantly against ignorance and quackery among the masses and follies of all sorts among the classes, *diagnosis,* not *drugging,* is our chief weapon of offence.

CHAUVINISM IN MEDICINE, IN AEQUANIMITAS, 283.

317. Evaluate your diagnoses without self-deception.

Begin early to make a threefold category—clear cases, doubtful cases, mistakes. And learn to play the game fair, no self-deception, no shrinking from the truth; mercy and consideration for the other man, but none for yourself, upon whom you have to keep an incessant watch.

THE STUDENT LIFE, IN AEQUANIMITAS, 412.

318. Absolute diagnoses are unsafe.

Absolute diagnoses are unsafe, and are made at the expense of the conscience.

BEAN WB. SIR WILLIAM OSLER: APHORISMS, 129.

319. Incorrect diagnoses lead to useless treatments.

Lack of systematic personal training in the methods of the recognition of disease leads to the misapplication of remedies, to long courses of treatment when treatment is useless, and so directly to that lack of confidence in our methods which is apt to place us in the eyes of the public on a level with empirics and quacks.

CHAUVINISM IN MEDICINE, IN AEQUANIMITAS, 283.

320. Missing the diagnosis causes a sore spot in the brain.

Use the knife and the cautery to cure the intumescence and moral necrosis which you will feel in the posterior parietal region, in Gall and Spurzheim's [18th century phrenologists] centre of self-esteem, where you will find a sore spot after you have made a mistake in diagnosis.

THE STUDENT LIFE, IN AEQUANIMITAS, 412.

321. Confessing ignorance is better than a hypothesis.

Frankly to confess ignorance is often wiser than to beat about the bush with a hypothetical diagnosis.

CAMAC CNB. COUNSELS AND IDEALS. BOSTON: HOUGHTON MIFFLIN, 2ND ED, 1929:214.

322. Never make a positive diagnosis.

Probability is the rule of life—especially under the skin. Never make a positive diagnosis.

CUSHING H. THE LIFE OF SIR WILLIAM OSLER, VOL. 1, 593.

323. Medical common sense is rare.

Common sense in matters medical is rare, and is usually in inverse ratio to the degree of education.

TEACHING AND THINKING, IN AEQUANIMITAS, 124.

324. Variability is the law of life.

Variability is the law of life, and as no two faces are the same, so no two bodies are alike, and no two individuals react alike and behave alike under the abnormal conditions which we know as disease.

ON THE EDUCATIONAL VALUE OF THE MEDICAL SOCIETY, IN AEQUANIMITAS, 331.

325. No two cases are alike.

As no two faces, so no two cases are alike in all respects, and unfortunately it is not only the disease itself which is so varied, but the subjects themselves have peculiarities which modify its action.

TEACHING AND THINKING, IN AEQUANIMITAS, 123.

326. Humans are variable.

As clinical observers, we study the experiments which Nature makes upon our fellow-creatures. These experiments, however, in striking contrast to those of the laboratory, lack exactness, possessing as they do a variability at once a despair and a delight—the despair of those who look for nothing but fixed laws in an art which is still deep in the sloughs of

Empiricism; the delight of those who find in it an expression of a universal law transcending, even scorning, the petty accuracy of test-tube and balance, the law that in man "the measure of all things," [from *Satires* by Horace (65-8 BC)] mutability, variability, mobility, are the very marrow of his being.

THE ARMY SURGEON, IN AEQUANIMITAS, 106.

327. *Be wary of diagnoses of exclusion.*

Adhesions are the refuge of the diagnostically destitute.

BEAN WB. SIR WILLIAM OSLER: APHORISMS, 144.

328. *It takes courage to make a prognosis.*

It takes courage to make a prognosis. Fulness of knowledge does not always bring confidence; the more one knows the more timidity may grow. The faculty which enables a man to look all round a question, to take a philosophical view of it, may be tempered with doubt, and an inability to reach a conclusion. A cocksure diagnosis and a positive prognosis may express the assurance of ignorance.

LUMLEIAN LECTURES ON ANGINA PECTORIS. LANCET 1910;1:973-7.

329. *The more the doctors, the sadder the prognosis.*

Can anything be more doleful than a procession of four or five doctors into the sick man's room?

MONTREAL MED J 1896;24:518-22.

Note-Taking

330. *Learn by a careful study of patients; wisdom requires experience.*

Upon young men just starting [in private practice] I would like to urge particularly to take careful notes of their cases, and to study each individual patient intelligently. Experience in any disease is not a measure of the number of cases seen; it is not a matter of mere accretion, of the adding fact to fact, this is knowledge. True experience brings more than knowledge; it brings wisdom, and this is a question of personal mental development.

ON THE STUDY OF PNEUMONIA. ST. PAUL MED J 1899;1:5-9.

331. *Note-taking is valuable.*

I wish I had time to speak of the value of note-taking. You can do nothing as a student in practice without it. Carry a small notebook which will fit into your waistcoat pocket, and never ask a new patient a question without notebook and pencil in hand.

THE STUDENT LIFE, IN AEQUANIMITAS, 411-2.

332. *Write down your observations.*

Don't trust your memory. Make notes. Write down your observations.

LONGCOPE WT. RANDOM RECOLLECTIONS OF WILLIAM OSLER, 1899-1918. ARCH INTERN MED 1949;84:93-103.

333. *Record your experiences.*

In a ten or fifteen years' service, travelling with seeing eyes and hearing ears, and carefully kept note-books, just think what a store-house of clinical material may be at the command of any one of you—material not only valuable in itself to the profession, but of infinite value to you personally in its acquisition, rendering you painstaking and accurate, and giving you, year by year, an increasing experience.

THE ARMY SURGEON, IN AEQUANIMITAS, 109.

334. Record what you have seen.

Record that which you have seen; make a note at the time; do not wait.

THAYER WS. OSLER THE TEACHER, IN OSLER AND OTHER PAPERS, 1.

335. Note and record the unusual.

Always note and record the unusual. Keep and compare your observations. Communicate or publish short notes on anything that is striking or new. Do not waste your time in compilations, but when your observations are sufficient, do not let them die with you. Study them, tabulate them, seek the points of contact which may reveal the underlying law. Some things can be learned only by statistical comparison. If you have the good fortune to command a large clinic, remember that one of your chief duties is the tabulation and analysis of the carefully recorded experience.

THAYER WS. OSLER THE TEACHER, IN OSLER AND OTHER PAPERS, 2.

5

Disease, Specific Illnesses, Lifestyle, Drugs

→ Disease

→ Specific Illnesses
- Cardiac Disease
- Infectious Disease
- Pneumonia
- Skin Disease
- Tuberculosis
- Venereal Disease
- Miscellaneous Diseases

→ Lifestyle
- Diet
- Exercise
- Vices

→ Drugs and Pharmaceutical Companies

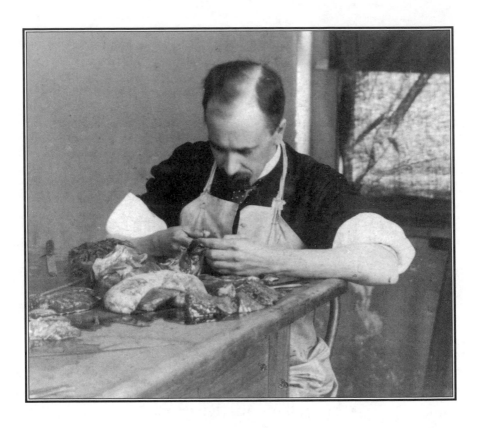

William Osler at the autopsy table at Blakely Hospital, Philadelphia, circa 1889.
(Courtesy of the Osler Library of the History of Medicine,
Montreal, Quebec, Canada.)

Disease, Specific Illnesses, Lifestyle, Drugs

Disease

336. Clinical judgment comes through experience.

We must know the natural course and tendencies of disease and be able to estimate the importance of complications and the indication of special symptoms which may arise. Experience alone can teach you this. Among the most trying duties of your early years in practice will be the weighing for anxious friends the probabilities of life and death; but in this respect, every year of careful study will strengthen your powers and add to your prognostic skill.

UNPUBLISHED DRAFT OF AN ADDRESS TO MEDICAL STUDENTS AT THE UNIVERSITY OF PENNSYLVANIA, 1885. PUBLISHED PRIVATELY BY THE OSLER LIBRARY, MCGILL UNIVERSITY, MONTREAL, 2006.

337. With disease, certainties become probabilities.

In taking up the study of disease, you leave the exact and certain for the inexact and doubtful and enter a realm in which to a great extent the certainties are replaced by probabilities.

UNPUBLISHED DRAFT OF AN ADDRESS TO MEDICAL STUDENTS AT THE UNIVERSITY OF PENNSYLVANIA, 1885. PUBLISHED PRIVATELY BY THE OSLER LIBRARY, MCGILL UNIVERSITY, MONTREAL, 2006.

338. Know pathology to appreciate disease in the living.

As a thorough acquaintance with normal anatomy is essential in studying the functions of the body in health, so is a knowledge of the organs and tissues of the body in disease an absolute necessity for the proper appreciation of the phenomena of disease during life.

UNPUBLISHED DRAFT OF AN ADDRESS TO MEDICAL STUDENTS AT THE UNIVERSITY OF PENNSYLVANIA, 1885. PUBLISHED PRIVATELY BY THE OSLER LIBRARY, MCGILL UNIVERSITY, MONTREAL, 2006.

339. Disease begins as a perversion of cell life.

The laws of cell growth and development are at the basis of all Physiology. Those modifications of nutrition which are abnormal and which we call disease also begin as perversions of cell life. Your subsequent conception of the intimate processes of disease will depend very much on the knowledge you obtain of the laws of cell life.

UNPUBLISHED DRAFT OF AN ADDRESS TO MEDICAL STUDENTS AT THE UNIVERSITY OF PENNSYLVANIA, 1885. PUBLISHED PRIVATELY BY THE OSLER LIBRARY, MCGILL UNIVERSITY, MONTREAL, 2006.

340. Knowledge makes possible cure or control of disease.

The whole life of the profession, whether moving in the units or expressed in its great institutions, is controlled to-day, as it ever has been controlled, by what we think of the nature of disease. Why is a right judgment on this one point the aim of medical education and of research—the be-all and the end-all of our efforts? Because upon correct knowledge depends the possibility of the control of disease, and upon our views of its nature the measures for its prevention or cure.

THE PATHOLOGICAL INSTITUTE OF A GENERAL HOSPITAL. GLASGOW MED J
1911;76:321-33.

341. No measure can compare with the alleviation of disease and suffering.

Measure as we may the progress of the world—intellectually in the growth and spread of education, materially in the application to life of all mechanical appliances, and morally in a higher standard of ethics between nation and nation, and between individuals, there is no one measure which can compare with the decrease of disease and suffering in man, woman and child.

MAN'S REDEMPTION OF MAN. NEW YORK: PAUL B. HOEBER, 1915:31.

342. Disease and pain are facts of life.

In the struggle for existence in which all life is engaged, disease and pain loom large as fundamental facts.

MAN'S REDEMPTION OF MAN. NEW YORK: PAUL B. HOEBER, 1915:9.

343. Look forward to peace and health.

Utopian as it may appear, we may look forward with hope to the day when the great enemies of our race shall be no more, when fever, war and pestilence shall cease to harass mankind.

THE STUDY OF THE FEVERS OF THE SOUTH. JAMA 1896;26:999-1000.

344. Medicine has three phases: recognize disease; discover its causes; prevent it.

Medicine proper has passed through three phases of activity—the recognition of disease and the means for its cure, the discovery of its causes, and the measures for its prevention.

THE SCHOOL OF PHYSIC, DUBLIN, IN MEN AND BOOKS, 28.

345. Medicine, ministry, and the law all share unsolvable problems.

There are incurable diseases in medicine, incorrigible vices in the ministry, insoluble cases in law.

BEAN WB. SIR WILLIAM OSLER: APHORISMS, 123.

346. The description of a disease and its manifestations may differ.

Early learn to appreciate the differences between the descriptions of disease and the manifestations of that disease in an individual—the difference between the composite portrait and one of the component pictures.

THE STUDENT LIFE, IN AEQUANIMITAS, 414.

347. Disease is complicated and variable in patients.

The problems of disease are more complicated and difficult than any others with which the trained mind has to grapple; the conditions in any given case may be unlike those in any other;...The science on which it is based is accurate and definite enough; the physics of a man's circulation are the physics of the waterworks of the town in which he lives, but once out of gear, you cannot apply the same rules for the repair of the one as of the other.

ON THE EDUCATION VALUE OF THE MEDICAL SOCIETY, IN AEQUANIMITAS, 331.

348. Understand the character and the manifestations of a disease.

In the consideration of a disease it is well, if possible, to start with a clear understanding, or at least some concise statement, of its nature, and of the characters of the manifestations by which it is recognized.

LECTURES ON ANGINA PECTORIS AND ALLIED STATES, 8.

349. Begin with a knowledge of the natural history of disease.

The fundamental law should be engrained that the starting point of all treatment is in a knowledge of the natural history of a disease.

THE RESERVES OF LIFE. ST. MARY'S HOSP GAZ 1907;13:95-8.

350. The numerical method of studying disease is self-evident.

To get an accurate knowledge of any disease it is necessary to study a large series of cases and to go into all the particulars—the conditions under which it is met, the subjects specially liable, the various symptoms, the pathological changes, the effects of drugs. This method, so simple, so self-evident, we owe largely to Louis [Pierre Charles Louis (1787-1872), Paris physician who invented the statistical method].

THE INFLUENCE OF LOUIS ON AMERICAN MEDICINE, IN AN ALABAMA STUDENT, 193.

351. Use guidelines for naming diseases.

"What's in a name?" may well be asked of the disorder under discussion, to which an unusual number of labels have been attached. The all important matter is to define as accurately as possible the condition named, according to the good rule laid down by Socrates: "Now, I have no objection to your giving names any significance you please if you will only tell me what you mean by them." [from *Charimedes* by Plato] If our knowledge does not permit to give a name according with the etiology of the disease, the rule should be to pick the one which seems least objectionable, taking priority and usage into account.

ANEMIA SPLENICA. TRANS ASSOC AM PHYS 1902;17:429-61.

352. The stages of recognition of a new disease are several.

It is interesting to follow the stages in the recognition of a new disease. Very rarely does it happen that at all points the description is so complete as at once to gain universal acceptance.... First a case here and there is reported as something unusual; in a year or two someone collects them and emphasizes the clinical features and perhaps names the disease. Then in rapid succession new cases are reported and we are surprised to find that it is by no means uncommon.

A CLINICAL LECTURE ON ERYTHRAEMIA. LANCET 1908;1:143-6.

353. Value the clinical-postmortem correlations.

In the investigation of disease a knowledge of the morbid phenomena observed during life and of the organic alterations found after death are inseparable. The teaching of the post-mortem room must supplement and illustrate the lessons of the ward.

NOTES ON THE MORBID ANATOMY OF PNEUMONIA. CAN MED SURG J 1884-85;13:596-605.

354. It is difficult to discern prognostic factors in diseases in which mortality is high.

The higher the mortality the more difficult it is to estimate in any disease the value of the various elements of prognosis.

ON CERTAIN FEATURES IN THE PROGNOSIS OF PNEUMONIA. AM J MED SCI 1897;
113:1-10.

355. More people are killed by hurry than disease.

Hurry? Never hurry—hurry is the devil. More people are killed by hurry than by disease.

OSBORNE M. RECOLLECTIONS OF SIR WILLIAM OSLER. IN ABBOTT ME (ED). SIR
WILLIAM OSLER MEMORIAL NUMBER. BULLETIN NO. IX OF THE INTERNATIONAL
ASSOCIATION OF MEDICAL MUSEUMS AND JOURNAL OF TECHNICAL METHODS.
MONTREAL: PRIVATELY PRINTED, 1926.

356. Take care of yourself.

Learn early to take the best possible care of the machine, never overdriving it, nor letting rust or dust collect in the bearings, and providing it with enough fuel to keep it going at a fair pace. Unlike any ordinary mechanism, the more you use it, the more, within limits, can you get out of it. Healthy action in a body out of which you can get plenty of work is the first great asset in the race, the most important part, perhaps, of life's reserves.

THE RESERVES OF LIFE. ST. MARY'S HOSP GAZ 1907;13:95-8.

Specific Illnesses

CARDIAC DISEASE

357. Treat the peripheral resistance, not the heart.

The difficulty is to keep the human irrigation plant free from weeds, the sud that chokes the capillary bed, through which it takes a greater force to drive the fluids. We too often tinker at the pump [heart] and the mains, instead of looking for the real seat of trouble in the fields.

BRIT MED J 1912;2:1733-7.

358. There are three stages of cardiac hypertrophy.

The course of any case of cardiac hypertrophy may be divided into three stages:

a. The period of development

b. The period of full compensation...during which the heart's vigor meets the requirements of the circulation.

c. The period of broken decompensation.

THE PRINCIPLES AND PRACTICE OF MEDICINE, 1ST EDITION, 1892, 634.

359. Life's tragedies are often arterial.

The tragedies of life are largely arterial.

DISEASES OF THE CIRCULATORY SYSTEM. IN OSLER W AND MCCRAE T (EDS). MODERN MEDICINE: ITS THEORY AND PRACTICE. PHILADELPHIA: LEA & FEBIGER, 1908:431.

360. Long life depends on your arteries.

Longevity is a vascular question.

Martin CF. Osler as a Clinician and Teacher. Can Med Assoc J, July 1920;82-6.

361. Modern life favors arteriosclerosis.

The conditions of modern life favor arteriosclerosis as a man is apt to work his body machine at high pressure and often takes less care of it than of his motor.

Diseases of the Circulatory System. In Osler W and McCrae T (eds). Modern Medicine: Its Theory and Practice. Philadelphia: Lea & Febiger, 1908:430.

362. Nature exacts retribution by arteriosclerosis.

Angeio-sclerosis, creeping on slowly but surely, "with no pace perceived," is the Nemesis through which Nature exacts retributive justice for the transgression of her laws—coming to one as an apoplexy, to another as an early Bright's disease, to a third as an aneurysm, and to a fourth as angina pectoris, too often slitting "the thin spun life" in the fifth decade, at the very time when success seems assured.

Lectures on Angina Pectoris and Allied States, 154.

363. Arterial disease develops at different rates in individuals.

There are two essential factors in arterio-sclerosis—the quality of the tubing and the way it is treated. The marvel is that any set of pipes could be constructed to stand the continuous strain to which for years the human blood vessels are subjected.... The contract calls for from sixty to eighty years of usage. Some hold out well, and even after ninety years are still fairly good, but the personal equation has always to be considered.

An Address of High Blood Pressure: Its Associations, Advantages, and Disadvantages. Brit Med J 1912;2:1733-7.

364. The cause of arteriosclerosis.

More commonly the arterio-sclerosis results from the bad use of good vessels.

THE PRINCIPLES AND PRACTICE OF MEDICINE, 848.

365. The pace of modern life causes premature arteriosclerosis.

Nothing is more certain than that the pace of modern life kills many prematurely through the complications of arterio-sclerosis. The keen, sharp business or professional man, year in, year out, giving his energies no rest, leading a life of high pressure, though a teetotaler and temperate in his diet, and a nonsmoker, may have so driven his machine that at 50 it is only fit to be scrapped.

AN ADDRESS OF HIGH BLOOD PRESSURE. BRIT MED J 1912;2:8.

366. Coronary arteries are vascular rivers of life.

The coronary arteries are the Abana and Pharpar of the vascular rivers, "lucid streams," which water the very citadel of life. [The Abana and the Pharpar are the two rivers of Damascus mentioned in the Bible.]

LECTURES ON ANGINA PECTORIS AND ALLIED STATES, 11.

367. Wise individuals develop coronary artery disease.

We may say of it [coronary disease] as Sydenham [Thomas Sydenham (1624-1689), English physician] did of the gout, that more wise men than fools are its victims.

LECTURES ON ANGINA PECTORIS AND ALLIED STATES, 21-2.

368. *The anterior descending is the artery of sudden death.*

This anterior branch is the important one in the morbid anatomy of the coronary arteries, since it is by far the most frequently found the seat of extensive sclerosis or of embolism or thrombosis. It may be called the *artery of sudden death.*

LECTURES ON ANGINA PECTORIS AND ALLIED STATES, 12.

369. *"Life struck sharp on Death" is due to coronary disease.*

An explanation of the awful suddenness—"Life struck sharp on Death" [from *Aurora Leigh* by Elizabeth Barrett Browning (1806-1861)]—is probably to be found in the arrest of the heart in fibrillary contraction.

LECTURES ON ANGINA PECTORIS AND ALLIED STATES, 33.

370. *Sudden death can be due to angina pectoris.*

A man in full health, in the prime of life, may be seized with a paroxysm of angina, and die within a few hours.

LECTURES ON ANGINA PECTORIS AND ALLIED STATES, 33-4.

371. *There is a sensation of imminent death with angina.*

There is an element peculiar to certain conditions of the heart, often associated with, but which cannot itself be properly characterized as pain—indeed, the patient often expressly states that it is not of the nature of physical pain—a sense of imminent dissolution, a mental anguish, which has been variously expressed by patients and writers as a pause in the operations of Nature, the very hand of death, *angor animi,* etc. This it is which constitutes the special feature in a majority of the cases of true angina.

LECTURES ON ANGINA PECTORIS AND ALLIED STATES, 9.

372. Osler's description of angina.

Angina pectoris…It is characterized by agonizing pain in the region of the heart and cramps in the left arm. The feelings vary from discomfort to agonizing sensations. There may be a terrible substernal pressure (dolor pectoris). Mental symptoms may be present. There is usually a feeling of impending death (angor animi). Vaso-motor phenomena occur producing paleness. The patient may even faint. The disease develops after the middle period of life…. Sudden death follows in a large percentage of cases…. Many of the sudden deaths you read of in healthy, vigorous men, especially at night, are due to angina pectoris.

PRATT JH: A YEAR WITH OSLER, 16-17.

373. Angina causes an anguish of mind.

One of the most distinguishing features of true angina is a consciousness on the part of the patient, in his anguish of mind, that the very citadel of life has been approached…. Subjects of the disease may truly be said to stand in jeopardy every hour, yet it is astonishing with what equanimity the affliction is endured.

LECTURES ON ANGINA PECTORIS AND ALLIED STATES, 139.

374. Anginal chest pain evokes a fear of dying.

For no man suffers the anguish of a severe paroxysm of angina without a consciousness of the nearness of the Angel of Death.

LECTURES ON ANGINA PECTORIS AND ALLIED STATES, 142.

375. The agony of angina pectoris is terrible.

The *attitude* during an attack is best described by the word immobile. If seized on the street, the patient grasps a lamp-post or leans against a wall, unable to stir until the agony has passed off.

LECTURES ON ANGINA PECTORIS AND ALLIED STATES, 51-2.

376. Characteristic events precipitate angina.

In true angina the patient can nearly always fix upon some provocation, as muscular effort, mental irritation, an attack of indigestion; whereas in pseudo-angina the attacks are much more apt to occur spontaneously, and rarely are excited by effort.

LECTURES ON ANGINA PECTORIS AND ALLIED STATES, 137.

377. Angina is difficult to diagnose.

One must be a professional Ulysses [Greek hero in Homer's *The Iliad* and *The Odyssey*] in craft and wisdom not sometimes to err in estimating the nature of an attack of severe heart pain. There is no group of cases so calculated to keep one in a condition of wholesome humility.

LECTURES ON ANGINA PECTORIS AND ALLIED STATES, 131.

378. Differentiate angina from functional chest pain.

In determining between a true and a false angina, the phenomena of the attack offer most valuable differential criteria. The character of the pain in pseudo-angina, while it may be very severe, rarely has the agonizing quality of true angina, and is seldom, if ever, associated with the sensation of impending death.

LECTURES ON ANGINA PECTORIS AND ALLIED STATES, 135-6.

379. The wrong diagnosis of coronary disease is a relief.

Successful treatment [of coronary disease] depends often upon correct diagnosis.... To a man who has felt that judgment has been given against him, the doom pronounced, and whose mind is haunted with the dread of sudden death, the assurance that the condition is functional and curable comes as a reprieve, and may be the one thing necessary to effect the cure.

LECTURES ON ANGINA PECTORIS AND ALLIED STATES, 143.

380. It is difficult to distinguish between different causes of stroke.

The chief difficulty in deciding upon a method of treatment [of stroke] is to determine whether the apoplexy is due to haemorrhage or to thrombosis or embolism.

THE PRINCIPLES AND PRACTICE OF MEDICINE, 980.

381. Missing an aortic aneurysm is humbling.

There is no disease more conducive to clinical humility than aneurysm of the aorta.

BEAN WB. SIR WILLIAM OSLER: APHORISMS, 138.

382. Endocarditis is difficult to diagnose.

Few diseases [endocarditis] present greater difficulties in the way of diagnosis, difficulties which in many cases are practically insurmountable…. The protean character of the malady, the latency of the cardiac symptoms, and the close simulation of other disorders, combine to render the detection peculiarly difficult.

GULSTONIAN LECTURES ON MALIGNANT ENDOCARDITIS. LANCET 1885;1:505-8.

383. Endocarditis may become chronic.

Endocarditis is always a serious lesion, if not immediately by loss of substance, etc., remotely by the sclerotic changes which it initiates, and which lead in a majority of the cases to retraction and insufficiency of the valve…. Nor is the term acute free of difficulties…there are cases in which the process is active and symptom-producing for eight, ten, twelve, or more months—an essentially chronic condition.

ACUTE ENDOCARDITIS. IN OSLER W AND MCCRAE T (EDS). MODERN MEDICINE: ITS THEORY AND PRACTICE. PHILADELPHIA: LEA & FEBIGER, 1908;4:133.

384. The diagnostic points of endocarditis.

The important points in the diagnosis are: the existence of a septic focus and a septic state as indicated by the temperature, the blood cultures, etc.; the presence of petechiae and embolic features, and the symptoms and physical signs pointing to a valvular lesion. Where the septic element dominates, the endocarditis is usually overlooked. When the cardiovascular features are well marked the diagnosis is usually made.

ACUTE ENDOCARDITIS. IN OSLER W AND MCCRAE T (EDS). MODERN MEDICINE: ITS
THEORY AND PRACTICE. PHILADELPHIA: LEA & FEBIGER, 1908;4:148.

385. A new murmur and embolus suggests endocarditis.

The development under observation of pronounced murmurs, particularly of aortic and regurgitant, is most suggestive of malignant endocarditis, and the occurrence of emboli would be a positive confirmation.

GULSTONIAN LECTURES ON MALIGNANT ENDOCARDITIS. LANCET 1885;1:505-8.

386. Endocarditis has an insidious course.

In the second great group, in which the vegetations form the focus of a chronic septicaemia, the diagnosis is by no means easy. The patients are the subjects of an old although often overlooked and well-compensated valve lesion. The fever begins insidiously.... Week after week, month after month, the daily rise of temperature may be the only feature, and, indeed, the patient may feel pretty well and be up and about for many weeks.

ACUTE ENDOCARDITIS. IN OSLER W AND MCCRAE T (EDS). MODERN MEDICINE: ITS
THEORY AND PRACTICE. PHILADELPHIA: LEA & FEBIGER, 1908;4:148.

387. Endocarditis may present with emboli.

In a considerable series of cases the history is somewhat as follows; the patient has, say, aortic valve disease, and is under treatment for failing compensation, when he begins to have slight irregular fever, an evening exacerbation of two or three degrees, some increase in cardiac pain, and a sense of restlessness and distress. Embolic phenomena may develop; a sudden hemiplegia; pain in the region of the spleen, and signs of enlargement of the organ; or there is pain in the back, with bloody urine. In other instances, peripheral embolism may take place, with gangrene of the foot or hand. There may be hebetude [apathy] or a low delirium. Instances such as these are extremely common; and while, in some, the process may be very intense, in others it is essentially chronic, and may last for weeks and months, so that the term malignant seems not at all applicable to them; still, in a large series of cases, all gradations can be seen between the most severe and the milder forms.

GULSTONIAN LECTURES ON MALIGNANT ENDOCARDITIS. LANCET 1885;1:459-64.

388. Profuse sweating is a frequent symptom of endocarditis.

Sweating [in endocarditis] is a very frequent symptom, and is worthy of special notice, from the peculiarly drenching character, which is…second only to ague, and usually far beyond the average mark of phthisis [tuberculosis] or pyaemia.

GULSTONIAN LECTURES ON MALIGNANT ENDOCARDITIS. LANCET 1885;1:459-64.

389. Description of Osler's nodes.

One of the most interesting features of the disease [endocarditis] and one to which very little attention has been paid is the occurrence of ephemeral spots of a painful nodular erythema, chiefly in the skin of the hands and feet.

CHRONIC INFECTIOUS ENDOCARDITIS. QUART J MED 1908-9;2:219-30.

390. Another description of Osler's nodes.

Painful subcutaneous nodules of a peculiar form may be present, not exactly like the fibroid nodules of rheumatic fever, but rather resembling minute emboli of the skin. The spots are painful, reddish, slightly raised, and disappear in a day or two.

> ACUTE ENDOCARDITIS. IN OSLER W AND MCCRAE T (EDS). MODERN MEDICINE: ITS
> THEORY AND PRACTICE. PHILADELPHIA: LEA & FEBIGER, 1908;4:148.

391. Petechiae are seen in endocarditis.

The occurrence of a rash [in endocarditis] has been described.... The most common form is the haemorrhagic, in the form of small petechiae.

> GULSTONIAN LECTURES ON MALIGNANT ENDOCARDITIS. LANCET 1885;1:459-64.

392. The skin and mucous membranes are the main entrance of bacterial endocarditis.

Practically in all cases the microorganisms gain entrance through the skin or mucous membranes.

> ACUTE ENDOCARDITIS. IN OSLER W AND MCCRAE T (EDS). MODERN MEDICINE: ITS
> THEORY AND PRACTICE. PHILADELPHIA: LEA & FEBIGER, 1908;4:138.

393. Endocarditis is an infectious process.

Briefly stated, the theory of acute endocarditis which at present prevails. . . is that it is in all its forms an essentially mycotic process; the local and constitutional effects being produced by the growth on the valves, and the transference to distant parts of microbes, which vary in character with the disease in which it develops.

> GULSTONIAN LECTURES ON MALIGNANT ENDOCARDITIS. LANCET 1885;1:505-8.

394. *The pathological changes of endocarditis with all their gradations are the result of the same process.*

Anatomically, there appear to be no very essential differences in the various forms of acute endocarditis. Between the small papillary excrescence and the huge fungating vegetation with destructive changes all gradations can be traced, and the last may be the direct outcome of the first; the two extremes indeed may be present in the same valve. They represent different degrees of intensity of one and the same process.

GULSTONIAN LECTURES ON MALIGNANT ENDOCARDITIS. LANCET 1885;1:416-8.

395. *The cardiac sites affected by endocarditis.*

Infective endocarditis is a valvular, rarely a mural, lesion, and on the valves the closure lines are points of election, viz., on the aortic cusps a little below the free edge and on the auriculoventricular valves the auricular faces, a little distance from the margin.... Malformations, as, for example, the edge of an imperforate septum, and valves which have sclerotic changes are especially prone to be attacked.

ACUTE ENDOCARDITIS. IN OSLER W AND MCCRAE T (EDS). MODERN MEDICINE: ITS THEORY AND PRACTICE. PHILADELPHIA: LEA & FEBIGER, 1908;4:134.

396. *Pericarditis is underdiagnosed.*

Probably no serious disease is so frequently overlooked [as pericarditis] by the practitioner. Post-mortem experience shows how often pericarditis is not recognized, or goes on to resolution and adhesion without attracting notice.

THE PRINCIPLES AND PRACTICE OF MEDICINE, 781.

397. *The diagnosis of pericarditis requires care.*

Pericarditis is diagnosed in proportion to the care of the examination.

BEAN WB. SIR WILLIAM OSLER: APHORISMS, 145.

398. Symptomatic pericardial tamponade should be drained.

When the effusion [in tuberculous pericarditis] reaches a certain grade, and the pulse is irregular and feeble, the color becoming bad, the respirations hurried, paracentesis should be performed, or, if necessary, the sac freely incised and drained.

TUBERCULOUS PERICARDITIS. AM J MED SCI 1893;105:20-37.

399. Osler's description of the murmur of mitral stenosis.

The time of the murmur [mitral stenosis] in the cardiac cycle and the quality—vibrating, rough, interrupted, and echoing—are associated with trouble at the mitral orifice. You may hear a similar murmur of blubbering quality secondary to aortic insufficiency but this never terminates in the sharp snappy first sound.

PRATT JH. A YEAR WITH OSLER, 95.

400. The difficulty of diagnosing mitral stenosis.

Mitral stenosis may be concealed under a quarter of a dollar. It is the most difficult of all heart diseases to diagnose.

BEAN WB. SIR WILLIAM OSLER: APHORISMS, 142.

401. The postural enhancement of the murmur of mitral valve prolapse.

As she sits upright in the chair the heart sounds at the apex and base loud and clear; no murmur. When she stands a loud systolic murmur is heard at the apex, high-pitched, somewhat musical, of maximum intensity in the fifth interspace.

ON A REMARKABLE HEART MURMUR, HEARD AT A DISTANCE FROM THE CHEST WALL.
CAN MED SURG J 1879;8:518-9.

402. The examination of aortic insufficiency.

Aortic insufficiency is the only valve lesion which we can recognize at sight. There is no other condition with which so distinctive a type of throbbing of the arteries is associated…. The diastolic murmur, and the visible collapsing pulse are pathognomonic.

DISEASES OF THE VALVES OF THE HEART. IN OSLER W AND MCCRAE T (EDS). MODERN MEDICINE: ITS THEORY AND PRACTICE. PHILADELPHIA: LEA AND FEBIGER, 1908;4:219.

403. The examination of tricuspid regurgitation.

From a careful observation of the jugular pulsation in the neck and careful auscultation over the precordia, there is seldom much doubt as to the presence or absence of tricuspid regurgitation.

DISEASES OF THE VALVES OF THE HEART. IN OSLER W AND MCCRAE T (EDS). MODERN MEDICINE: ITS THEORY AND PRACTICE. PHILADELPHIA: LEA AND FEBIGER, 1908;4:245.

404. Description of functional heart disease.

The condition is comparable to the irritable heart mentioned by Da Costa [Jacob Da Costa (1833-1900), Philadelphia physician and teacher] as occurring in military life, particularly among young recruits…. The cases of irritable heart, occurring as a result of neurasthenia, are nearly twice as frequent in females as in men. They are accompanied by mental distress, debility, nervous dyspepsia, and, in women, uterine disease. There is sometimes a peculiar vaso-motor disturbance, causing flushing…. A feeling of impending death is a frequent and most distressing symptom in some cases.

THE IRRITABLE HEART OF CIVIL LIFE. CAN MED SURG J 1887;15:617-9.

405. Do not squander heartbeats.

Do not squander heartbeats in cardiac disease—live within your income.

BEAN WB. SIR WILLIAM OSLER: APHORISMS, 100.

406. Varicose veins are hereditary.

Varicose veins are the result of an improper selection of grandparents.

BEAN WB. SIR WILLIAM OSLER: APHORISMS, 146.

407. Anemia can make heart failure worse.

The anaemia of heart disease . . .The comfort of such patients is in direct proportion to their corpuscular richness, and without any apparent increase in the valve mischief, a reduction in the ratio of the corpuscles is followed by shortness of breath, palpitation, and signs of heart-failure.

ON THE USE OF ARSENIC IN CERTAIN FORMS OF ANAEMIA. THERAPEUTIC GAZ
(DETROIT) 1886;2:741-6.

408. Palpitations are common in emotional states.

There are cases in which complaint is made of the most distressing palpitation and sensations of throbbing, in which the physical examination reveals a regularly acting heart, the sensations being entirely subjective.... It is a very common symptom in hysteria and neurasthenia.

THE PRINCIPLES AND PRACTICE OF MEDICINE, 649.

409. Osler's sign of pseudohypertension.

It may be difficult to estimate how much of the hardness and firmness [of the radial artery] is due to the tension of the blood within the vessel, and how much to the thickening of the wall. If, for example, when the radial is compressed with the index-finger the artery can be felt beyond the point of compression, its walls are sclerosed.

THE PRINCIPLES AND PRACTICE OF MEDICINE, 668.

410. Cardiac hypertrophy is often well tolerated.

Hypertrophy [of the heart]...is not necessarily accompanied by symptoms. So admirable is the adjusting power of the heart that, for example, an advancing stenosis of aortic or mitral orifice may for years be perfectly equalized by a progressive hypertrophy, and the subject of the affection be happily unconscious of the existence of heart trouble.

THE PRINCIPLES AND PRACTICE OF MEDICINE, 587.

411. Capillaries are the middleman of life.

In the capillary lake into which the arterial stream widens the current slows and the pressure lessens...In the brief fraction of a second, and in a short quarter to three-quarters of a millimetre of space, the business of life is transacted, for here is the mart or exchange in which the raw and the manufactured articles from the intestinal and hepatic shops are spread out for sale. The endothelial capillary cell is not a simple dead membrane under the laws of diffusion, but has an active selective power. Playing the part of the middleman, it is everywhere a fee trader in the bread stuff of life, oxygen, but a strong protectionist in certain commodities. Thus the renal capillary cell trades in waters, salts, urea, and uric acid, but has a high tariff wall against proteins and sugars. In the secretory glands the selective capacity of the capillary wall must be of the first importance, as here the middleman and the retailer are cheek by jowl, and their shops abut, back to back, opening to different streets. These retail shops, represented by the gland and body cells of the capillary areas, do a roaring trade, partly in common commodities—water, oxygen, salts—and partly in special goods made up on the spot for the use of the body. Each cell, factory as well as shop, collects a great deal of dust and rubbish, and special provision is made for getting rid of this, part being dumped back into the common river, and part into a special lymphatic drainage system, which keeps the irrigation fields free from weeds and dirt. The transactions which take place between the middleman (the capillary cell), the factory and shop-people (in the gland or body cell), and the sanitary department (represented by the lymph circulation), are regulated in part by the laws of diffusion and osmosis, and partly by the cell specialists (enzymes of various sorts), some of which, for example, enable the liver cells to make bile, others to make glycogen.

AN ADDRESS ON HIGH PRESSURE. BRIT MED J 1912;2:1.

INFECTIOUS DISEASE

412. The physician's first responsibility is to warn the public quickly.

The welfare of an entire community may depend on the early recognition of the nature of the disease. With an outbreak at our doors, the physician will scrutinize sharply all dubious cases, and in a natural anxiety to protect the patient and his family from trouble and inconvenience, will remember also the larger obligation to do all in his power to prevent the spread of one of the most formidable of human scourges [cholera].

OSLER W. NOTES ON THE DIAGNOSIS AND TREATMENT OF CHOLERA. MEDICAL NEWS [PHILADELPHIA] 1892; 61:290-291.

413. The treatment and prevention of infectious disease is a boon to humanity.

It is worthy of comment that three of the greatest benefits conferred on mankind—beside which it would be hard to name three of equal importance—have been in connection with the fevers: The introduction of cinchona, the discovery of vaccination and the announcement of the principle of asepsis.

THE STUDY OF THE FEVERS OF THE SOUTH. JAMA 1896;26:999-1000.

414. Osler's condemnation of anti-vaccinationists.

I would like to issue a Mount Carmel-like [mountain in Israel] challenge to any ten unvaccinated priests of Baal [a false god or idol]. I will take ten selected vaccinated persons, and help in the next severe epidemic, with ten unvaccinated persons (if available!). I should choose three Members of Parliament, three anti-vaccination doctors, if they could be found, and four anti-vaccination propagandists. And I will make this promise—neither to jeer or to jibe when they catch the disease, but to look after them as brothers; and for the three or four who are certain to die I will try to arrange the funerals with all the pomp and ceremony of an anti-vaccination demonstration.

MAN'S REDEMPTION OF MAN. NEW YORK: PAUL B. HOEBER, 1915:46-7.

415. Fever (infectious disease) is humanity's worst enemy.

Humanity has but three great enemies: Fever, famine and war; of these by far the greatest, by far the most terrible, is fever.

THE STUDY OF THE FEVERS OF THE SOUTH. JAMA 1896;26:999-1000.

416. Determining the etiology of infections during the late 19th century was a great achievement.

One of the great facts in the history of the past century has been the remarkable increase in our knowledge of the infectious diseases.

THE PROBLEM OF TYPHOID FEVER IN THE UNITED STATES. MED NEWS [NEW YORK] 1899;74:225-9.

417. Improved sanitation has a major impact on infectious diseases.

Sixty years of sanitary reform have swept away typhus and cholera and have restricted yellow fever within narrow areas; we have learned how to fight tuberculosis and diphtheria, and in a hundred other ways the prevalence of the infectious disorders has been lessened. One demonstration stands out in clear relief above all others—with a clean soil and pure water typhoid fever disappears.

THE PROBLEM OF TYPHOID FEVER IN THE UNITED STATES. MED NEWS [NEW YORK] 1899;74:225-9.

418. Infectious diseases are often critical during times of war.

From the days of Homer, Apollo [Greek god of prophecy, medicine, music, and poetry], the far darter, has been a much more formidable foe than his colleague Mars [god of war]. With the two in conjunction unspeakable woes afflict the sons of men. In this great strait David, you remember, chose three days of pestilence as the equivalent of three months' military disaster. To-day [World War I] the front of Mars is wrinkled, the world is at war, and the problem for the children of Aesculapius is to keep grandfather Apollo from taking a hand in the fray. In this game another member of the family, Hygeia [goddess of health], holds the trump card and gives victory to the nation that can keep a succession of healthily efficient men in the field.

THE WAR AND TYPHOID FEVER. BRIT MED J 1914;2:909-13.

419. Bacillary dysentery has been a great scourge of armies.

Dysentery is one of the great camp diseases, and has been more destructive to armies than powder and shot.

THE PRINCIPLES AND PRACTICE OF MEDICINE, 243.

420. Combating plague requires resources and organization.

Wherever plague exists an organized staff, an intelligent policy, and a long purse are needed.

THE PRINCIPLES AND PRACTICE OF MEDICINE, 242.

421. Physicians should promote public health by early recognition of communicable disease.

The welfare of an entire community may depend on the early recognition of the nature of the disease. With an outbreak at our doors, so to speak, the physician will scrutinize sharply all dubious cases, and in a nat-

ural anxiety to protect the patient and his family from trouble and inconvenience, will remember also the larger obligation to do all in his power
to prevent the spread of one of the most formidable of human scourges
[cholera].

NOTES ON THE DIAGNOSIS AND TREATMENT OF CHOLERA. MED NEWS [PHILADELPHIA]
1892;61:290-1.

422. State Boards of Health should have more support.

Many of the State Boards of Health need a more efficient organization;
all need a larger annual appropriation. A bureau of public health should
form an integral department of each State government, with which civic,
county, township, town, and village boards should be in close organic
affiliation. The salaries of the health officers should be changed from the
beggarly pittance, almost the rule, to sums which would warrant a
demand on the part of the public that such officials should have modern
training in sanitary science.

THE PROBLEM OF TYPHOID FEVER IN THE UNITED STATES. MED NEWS [NEW YORK]
1899;74:225-9.

423. Physicians should be concerned not only about individual patients but also about public health.

Our ways, thank God, are not Nature's. Indulge as we may in speculation on the improvement of the race, in practice we care nothing for the
species, only for the individual. Reversing Nature's method, we are careless of the type, careful only of the single life. Year by year unwilling wit-
nesses of an appalling sacrifice, as fruitless as it is astounding, year by year
we physicians sit at the bed-sides of thousands upon thousands, chiefly
of youths and maidens, whose lives are offered up on the altars of
Ignorance and Neglect.

THE PROBLEM OF TYPHOID FEVER IN THE UNITED STATES. MED NEWS [NEW YORK]
1899;74:225-9.

424. Food safety is an important public health concern.

In the interests of public health, it is a matter of great importance that the food supply of cities should undergo strict supervision, with a view of excluding possible sources of disease.

AN INVESTIGATION INTO THE PARASITES IN THE PORK SUPPLY OF MONTREAL. CAN MED
SURG J 1882-1883;11:325-36.

425. The prevalence of typhoid fever correlates with sanitation.

The responsibility for the widespread prevalence of the disease [typhoid fever] rests directly upon the wanton carelessness of the people. God's own country, with man's own backyard, and the devil's own cesspools expresses existing situations. A three-fold duty devolves upon the members of our profession: First, to preach cleanliness! cleanliness! cleanliness!!!; secondly, to give a local and willing support to the State health officials; and thirdly, to regard every case of typhoid fever as a center and possible source of further infection.

THE PROBLEM OF TYPHOID FEVER IN THE UNITED STATES. MED NEWS [NEW YORK]
1899;74:225-9.

426. Germs cause infectious diseases.

If the changes in fermentation are due to minute living organisms, why should not the same tiny creatures make the changes which occur in the body in putrid or suppurative diseases?

THE PATHOLOGICAL INSTITUTE OF A GENERAL HOSPITAL. GLASGOW MED J
1911;76:321-33.

427. *Influenza is easy to recognize in the epidemic setting.*

During a pandemic [of influenza] the cases offer but slight difficulty. The profoundness of the prostration, out of all proportion to the intensity of the disease, is one of the most characteristic features.

THE PRINCIPLES AND PRACTICE OF MEDICINE, 155.

428. *Herpes zoster is extremely painful.*

In herpes [zoster] the pain may be very persistent. Patients have committed suicide on account of the pain of intercostal neuralgia.

PRATT JH. A YEAR WITH OSLER, 38.

429. *Tetanus can cause extreme hyperthermia.*

Tetanus more often than any other infection has a fever as high as 110-112° F.

PRATT JH. A YEAR WITH OSLER, 100.

430. *Secondary infections are often the immediate cause of death.*

There is truth in the paradoxical statement that persons rarely die of the disease with which they suffer. Secondary, *terminal,* infections carry off many of the incurable cases.

THE PRINCIPLES AND PRACTICE OF MEDICINE, 218.

431. *Whooping cough is terrible to behold.*

The child [with whooping cough] knows for a few moments when the attack is coming on, and tries in every way to check it, but failing to do so, runs terrified to the nurse or mother to be supported, or clutches anything near by. Few diseases are more painful to witness.

THE PRINCIPLES AND PRACTICE OF MEDICINE, 150.

432. *The gametocytes of Plasmodium falciparum are usually crescent-shaped.*

The form [malaria hematozoa] was usually that of a beautiful crescent, with rounded or gently tapering ends; but the degree of curvature was variable, and many forms were almost straight. The length is about double that of the width of a red corpuscle, sometimes more. They are not attached, and they never show any motion. Joining the ends of the crescents—or, more correctly, at a little distance from the points—a narrow line can often be seen on the concave margin. This, with the peculiar form, makes these bodies very easily recognizable in the blood, even when closely surrounded by the corpuscles.

AN ADDRESS ON THE HAEMATOZOA OF MALARIA. BRIT MED J 1887;1:556-62.

433. *Meningococcus is of low virulence but can be nasty.*

The meningococcus is a germ of low virulence, widely spread in the community, and of intense virulence in an individual once it has passed the portals of protection. It is doubtless carried from one person to another, not necessarily from patient to patient, as nurses, doctors, and attendants are very rarely attacked, but in a large proportion the germ is transmitted by a healthy carrier.

OSLER W. CEREBRO-SPINAL FEVER IN CAMPS AND BARRACKS. BRIT MED J 1915;
1:189-90.

434. The battle of the host versus infectious organisms.

If victory remains with the invaders the organisms pervade the affected part, multiply, and induce conditions incompatible with the life of the part, or perhaps with the life of the entire organism. If the battle is with the host, the parasites are destroyed, perhaps not without loss, but the normal state is gradually restored.

ON PHAGOCYTES. MED NEWS [PHILADELPHIA] 1889;54:421-5.

435. The best disinfectants.

Soap and water and common sense are the best disinfectants.

BEAN WB. SIR WILLIAM OSLER: APHORISMS, 134.

436. Lymph nodes imprison invaders.

A scraping from any moderately pigmented lymph gland shows that the chief part of its carbon load is warehoused (so to speak) in protoplasm, the granules lie for the most part imbedded free in a connective tissue matrix. Here the struggle is practically over, and though not a victory, yet the compromise which has been made is the best which could possibly be effected. The sharp irritating particles have been placed in position in which they could do the least harm, and, though not expelled, have been safely imprisoned.

ON PHAGOCYTES. MED NEWS [PHILADELPHIA] 1889;54:393-6.

PNEUMONIA

437. Pneumonia is a leading cause of death.

One of the most widespread and fatal of all acute diseases, pneumonia has become the "Captain of the Men of Death," to use the phrase applied by John Bunyan [(1628-1688), from *The Life and Death of Mr. Badman*] to consumption [tuberculosis].

THE PRINCIPLES AND PRACTICE OF MEDICINE, 165.

438. Pneumonia can be the "old person's friend."

Pneumonia may well be called the friend of the aged. Taken off by it in an acute, short, not often painful illness, the old man escapes those "cold gradations of decay" so distressing to himself and to his friends.

THE PRINCIPLES AND PRACTICE OF MEDICINE, 165.

439. Patients with lobar pneumonia have a typical appearance.

When seen on the second or third day, the picture in typical pneumonia is more distinctive than that presented by any other acute disease. The patient lies flat in bed, often on the affected side; the face is flushed, particularly one or both cheeks; the breathing is hurried, accompanied often with a short expiratory grunt; the alae nasi dilate with each inspiration; herpes is usually present on the lips or nose; the eyes are bright, the expression is anxious, and there is a frequent short cough which makes the patient wince and hold his side. The expectoration is blood-tinged and extremely tenacious.

THE PRINCIPLES AND PRACTICE OF MEDICINE, 172.

440. Fatal cases of pneumonia often have subtle manifestations.

Many of the cases [of pneumonia] which show the most profound toxaemia present variations from the typical picture; thus there may be no cough, no expectoration, very slight fever, and no leukocytosis.

ON CERTAIN FEATURES IN THE PROGNOSIS OF PNEUMONIA. AM J MED SCI 1897;11(NEW SERIES):1-10.

441. Mortality in pneumonia correlates with toxemia.

The toxaemia outweighs all other elements in the prognosis of pneumonia; to it (in a gradual failure of strength or more rarely in a sudden death, as in the cases given) is due in great part the terrible mortality from this common disease, and unhappily against it we have as yet no reliable measures at our disposal.

On Certain Features in the Prognosis of Pneumonia. Am J Med Sci 1897:11(new series):1-10.

442. Pneumonia may be serious in certain groups.

Pneumonia remains now, as then, the most serious acute disease with which physicians have to deal; serious because it attacks the old, the feeble, and the drunkard—persons who are not in a condition to withstand the sudden, sharp onset of the malady. But pneumonia is now, as it was formerly, a comparatively safe affection in healthy adults, easily managed, and with a low death-rate.

Has the Mortality in Pneumonia Increased? Med Rec [New York] 1888;34:604.

Skin Disease

443. Scleroderma is a shrinking skin of steel.

In its more aggravated forms diffuse scleroderma is one of the most terrible of all human ills. Like Tithonus [a Greek mythological hero who was granted immortality but not eternal youth. He was the subject of a poem by Tennyson (1809-1892).] to "wither slowly" and like him to be "beaten down and marred and wasted" until one is literally a mummy, encased in an evershrinking, slowly contracting skin of steel, is a fate not pictured in any tragedy, ancient or modern.

On Diffuse Scleroderma. J Cutan & Genitourin Dis 1898;16:49.

444. Scleroderma produces a mummy.

The hands [in scleroderma] are converted into rigid, immobile organs. In severe cases the unfortunate victim is as though he had been put in the fabled shirt of Nessus [the bloody shirt of a centaur killed by Hercules for trying to carry off his wife], which had gradually contracted upon him. The back is rigid, the neck is fixed, and he may resemble a frozen corpse or a mummy, without the power of motion, save in eyes and tongue, which alone gives witness to remaining life.

DIFFUSE SCLERODERMA; ERYTHROMELALGIA. IN MODERN MEDICINE: ITS THEORY AND PRACTICE, 3RD ED. PHILADELPHIA: LEA & FEBIGER, 1913-15:1019.

445. Description of hereditary hemorrhagic telangiectasia.

On the skin of the nose, of the cheeks and of the upper lip there were numerous small red spots due to dilatation of superficial vessels of the skin. Similar small telangiectases were seen on the internal surfaces of the lips, the cheeks, the tongue, and on the soft palate.

ON A FAMILY FORM OF RECURRING EPISTAXIS, ASSOCIATED WITH MULTIPLE TELANGIECTASES OF THE SKIN AND MUCOUS MEMBRANES. JOHNS HOPKINS HOSP BULL 1901;12:333-7.

446. Bleeding manifestations of hemorrhagic telangiectasia.

The disease [hereditary telangiectasia] is one of very serious character, as the bleedings are often of great severity, and in some of the cases have recurred with such frequency that a state of chronic anaemia has been produced.... In the great majority of the cases the bleeding is from the nose, and has the usual character of epistaxis. In other instances the blood comes from spots on the lips, the tongue, gums, and mucous membrane of the palate.

ON MULTIPLE HEREDITARY TELANGIECTASES WITH RECURRING HEMORRHAGES. QUART J MED 1907-08;1:53-8.

447. The structure and location of angiomata.

Angiomata are very peculiar and remarkable structures, in which I have been interested for many years…The spider angioma, formed by a) three or four dilated veins, which converge to and join a central vessel; or b) which unite at a central bright red nodule projecting a little beyond the skin. They are very common, and doctors are often consulted about their presence on the face.

ON A FAMILY FORM OF RECURRING EPISTAXIS, ASSOCIATED WITH MULTIPLE
TELANGIECTASES OF THE SKIN AND MUCOUS MEMBRANES. JOHNS HOPKINS HOSP BULL
1901;12:333-7.

448. Conditions in which naevi and telangiectases occur.

For many years I have been interested in the naevi and small telangiectatic spots which one sees so frequently in the routine examination of patients. Their increase as age advances, their peculiar distribution, their temporary character in young persons, the association with cirrhosis of the liver, the possible association with internal carcinoma, the occasional eruptive-like outbreak in jaundice, the remarkable hereditary form associated with epistaxis,…the presence of the spider-naevi in scleroderma, and their occurrence in the scar of X-ray burns.

ON TELANGIECTASIS CIRCUMSCRIPTA UNIVERSALIS. JOHNS HOPKINS HOSP BULL
1907;18:401-3.

449. Liver disease as a basis for some angiomata.

Angiomata have a curious relationship with affections of the liver. In cirrhosis, in cancer, in chronic jaundice from gallstones spider angiomata may appear on the face and other parts.

ON A FAMILY FORM OF RECURRING EPISTAXIS, ASSOCIATED WITH MULTIPLE
TELANGIECTASES OF THE SKIN AND MUCOUS MEMBRANES. JOHNS HOPKINS HOSP BULL
1901;12:333-7.

450. The relationship of spider nevi and hepatic cirrhosis.

The most interesting association of the spider naevus is with cirrhosis of the liver. In no other condition may we watch the development of such remarkable telangiectases.

ON MULTIPLE HEREDITARY TELANGIECTASES WITH RECURRING HEMORRHAGES.
QUART J MED 1907-08;1:53-8.

451. Description of common cherry angiomas.

The small nodular forms [now usually called cherry angiomas]...may be congenital, and there are few bodies on which they are not seen, but with the patches of pigmentation and the yellow, plaque-like warts [seborrheic keratoses] they form common senile changes in the skin of every one above sixty years of age.

ON MULTIPLE HEREDITARY TELANGIECTASES WITH RECURRING HEMORRHAGES.
QUART J MED 1907-08;1:53-8.

452. Principal manifestations of angioneurotic edema.

Definition [angioneurotic edema]—Localized swellings of the skin and subcutaneous tissues of the face and limbs, appearing spontaneously, and lasting from a few hours to a day or two. The mucous membranes of the lips, pharynx, larynx, gastro-intestinal canal, and genitals may be simultaneously involved, or they may be affected alone. The lesions in the skin are usually painless, but may be associated with itching and a sense of tension. Recurrences are the rule, and the swellings may appear at intervals throughout life. The affection may occur in many generations, and in many members of a family. In the majority of cases it is not serious, but the gastro-intestinal form causes severe colic, and in a few instances death has been caused by oedema of the glottis. The affection is closely related to urticaria.

ANGIONEUROTIC OEDEMA: QUINCKE'S DISEASE. IN OSLER W AND MCCRAE T (EDS).
MODERN MEDICINE: ITS THEORY AND PRACTICE. PHILADELPHIA: LEA & FEBIGER,
1909;6:648-64.

453. Clinical description of angioneurotic edema.

[On angioneurotic edema] The hands, face, and genitals, are most frequently attacked. Itching, heat, and redness often precede the outbreak. In many cases the patient also had urticaria.

HEREDITARY ANGIO-NEUROTIC OEDEMA. AM J MED SCI 1888:95:362-7.

454. Blood supply to the skin can change rapidly in Raynaud's disease.

The sudden blush of shame, the instantaneous pallor of fear, indicate the extraordinary rapidity of action, and illustrate, moreover, the extremes of vascularity in the skin.

VASOMOTOR AND TROPHIC DISORDERS: RAYNAUD'S DISEASE. IN OSLER W AND MCCRAE
T (EDS). MODERN MEDICINE: ITS THEORY AND PRACTICE. PHILADELPHIA: LEA &
FEBIGER, 1909:625-47.

455. Osler's description of systemic lupus erythematosus.

By exudative erythema is understood a disease of unknown etiology with polymorphic skin lesions—hyperaemia, oedema, and hemorrhage—arthritis occasionally, and a variable number of visceral manifestations, of which the most important are gastro-intestinal crises, endocarditis, pericarditis, acute nephritis, and hemorrhage from the mucous surfaces. Recurrence is a special feature...and attacks may come on...even throughout a long period of years.

ON THE VISCERAL MANIFESTATIONS OF ERYTHEMA EXUDATIVUM MULTIFORME. AM J
MED SCI 1895;110:629-46.

456. Polycythemia can cause a striking appearance.

The first case [polycythemia] I saw presented remarkable alterations in this respect. In the hot summer days he was "red as a rose" and looked bursting with blood and in the winter he became blue as indigo.

A CLINICAL LECTURE ON ERYTHRAEMIA. LANCET 1908;1:143-6.

457. Osler's description of polycythemia.

[The cyanosis] is most marked about the face and hands…but in both of my patients the skin of the entire body was of a dusky blue…. The viscidity [of the blood] is greatly increased. All observers have remarked not only upon the unusually dark, but upon the thick and sticky character of the blood drop. An extraordinary polycythaemia is a special feature of the affection…. In seven of the nine cases the spleen was enlarged. In four of these the enlargement may be termed great, reaching nearly to the navel.

CHRONIC CYANOSIS WITH POLYCYTHAEMIA AND ENLARGED SPLEEN: A NEW CLINICAL
ENTITY. AM J MED SCI 1903;126:187-201.

TUBERCULOSIS

458. Tubercle bacilli ride coal-polluted air.

Huge blocks of coal that would grace the doorstep of any multimillionaire coal dealer as a sign are carried into the lungs from our coal-polluted air, and tubercle bacilli ride in on coal-black chargers three abreast. Coal barges equal to those on the Susquehanna are constantly passing through unbroken mucosa and along lymph ducts to the bronchial lymph nodes.

BEAN WB. SIR WILLIAM OSLER: APHORISMS, 135.

459. Tuberculosis is a major scourge of humanity.

Tuberculosis is the most universal scourge of the human race. It prevails more particularly in the large cities and wherever the population is massed together.

THE PRINCIPLES AND PRACTICE OF MEDICINE, 284.

460. The treatment of tuberculosis requires a rigid regimen.

A rigid regimen, a life of rules and regulations, a dominant will on the part of the doctor, willing obedience on the part of the patient and friends—these, with the conditions we have discussed, are necessary in the treatment of pulmonary tuberculosis.

THE HOME TREATMENT OF CONSUMPTION. MARYLAND MED J 1900;43:8-12.

461. Patients with tuberculosis should not be treated as outcasts.

Tuberculosis patients should not be looked upon as social outcasts, to their own great distress and to the alarm of their families. For this feeling there is no justification. So long as a patient with tuberculosis takes the proper precautions there is no risk in close contact. If you are afraid of taking consumption, and desire a place of safety free from the germs of the disease, live in a first-class sanatorium, where fewer germs are scattered about than in the cities.

WHAT THE PUBLIC CAN DO IN THE FIGHT AGAINST TUBERCULOSIS. OXFORD: HORACE HART, 1909.

462. It is difficult to correlate lung capacity with survival.

It is difficult to say how much breathing-area is needed to maintain life. That a man can get along with very little, if the removal takes place gradually, is shown by cases of progressive tuberculosis of the lungs.

On Certain Features in the Prognosis of Pneumonia. Am J Med Sci 1897;11:1-10.

Venereal Disease

463. Know the manifestations of syphilis.

Know syphilis in all its manifestations and relations, and all other things clinical will be added unto you.

Bean WB. Sir William Osler: Aphorisms, 133.

464. Syphilis has many manifestations.

Syphilis, which begins its pathological existence as a modest, inactive Hunterian chancre, soon enters upon a career that is unsurpassed for the inclusiveness and variety of its manifestations. There is no organ in the body, nor any tissue in the organs, which syphilis does not invade: and it is therefore manifestly difficult to speak, at least at all concisely, of the pathology of the disease; just as it is almost impossible to describe its clinical symptoms without mentioning almost every symptom of every disease known.

Syphilis (with J.W. Churchman). Modern Medicine: Its Theory and Practice. Philadelphia: Lea Brothers, 1907;3:436-521.

465. Syphilis affects persons in all walks of life.

Syphilis is common in the community, and is no respecter of age, sex, or station in life.

THE PRINCIPLES AND PRACTICE OF MEDICINE, 278.

466. Gonorrhoea is a major cause of morbidity.

As a cause of ill-health and disability the gonococcus occupies a position of the very first rank among its fellows. While the local lesion is too often thought to be trifling, its singular obstinacy, in the possibilities of permanent sexual damage to the individual himself and still more in the "grisly troop" which may follow in its train, gonorrhoeal infection does not fall very far short of syphilis in importance.

THE PRINCIPLES AND PRACTICE OF MEDICINE, 281

467. Gonorrhea often sterilizes women.

The gonococcus is not a great destroyer of life.... But the gonococcus is the greatest known preventer of life—in fact, one of its cruel properties is to sterilize a very considerable proportion of its hosts. To realize the ravages of gonorrhoea, do not consult the Blue-books or the text-books, but study the reports of the gynaecological clinics and hospital for diseases of women.

THE ANTI-VENEREAL CAMPAIGN. TRANS MED SOC LONDON 1917;11:290-315.

468. Venereal diseases are a public menace.

It is appalling to contemplate the frightful train of miseries which a single diseased woman may entail, not alone on her associates, but on scores of the innocent—whose bitter cry should make the opponents of legislation feel that any measures of restriction, any measures of registration, would be preferable to the present disgraceful condition, which makes of some Christian cities open brothels and allows the purest homes to be invaded by the most loathsome of all diseases.

MEDICINE IN THE NINETEENTH CENTURY, IN AEQUANIMITAS, 252-3.

469. Sexual abstinence is the best prevention of sexually transmitted disease.

Personal purity is the prophylaxis which we, as physicians, are especially bound to advocate. Continence may be a hard condition (to some harder than to others), but it can be borne, and it is our duty to urge this lesson upon young and old who seek our advice in matters sexual. Certainly it is better, as St. Paul says, to marry than to burn, but if the former is not feasible there are other altars than those of Venus upon which a young man may light fires. He may practice at least two of the five means by which, as the physician Rondibilis counselled Panurge [from *Gargantua and Pantagruel* by Rabelais (1494-1553)], carnal concupiscence may be cooled and quelled—hard work of body and hard work of mind.

THE PRINCIPLES AND PRACTICE OF MEDICINE, 278-9.

470. Control your sexual passions.

Idleness is the mother of lechery; and a young man will find that absorption in any pursuit will do much to cool passions which, though natural and proper, cannot in the exigencies of our civilization always obtain natural and proper gratification.

THE PRINCIPLES AND PRACTICE OF MEDICINE, 279.

MISCELLANEOUS DISEASES

471. Osler's original description of the Parkinsonian tremor as pill-rolling.

The tremor is usually marked in the hands, and the thumb and forefinger display a motion made in the act of rolling a pill.

THE PRINCIPLES AND PRACTICE OF MEDICINE, 1043.

472. Friends recognize jaundice.

Jaundice is a disease that your friends diagnose.

BEAN WB. SIR WILLIAM OSLER: APHORISMS, 144.

473. Judicious exercise is useful in patients with neurasthenia.

During ordinary life nervous people should, during some portion of each day, pay rational attention to the body. Cold baths, swimming, exercises in the gymnasium, gardening, golf, lawn tennis, cricket, hunting, shooting, rowing, sailing, and bicycling are of value in maintaining the general nutrition. Such exercises are, of course, to be recommended only to individuals physically equal to them. If neurasthenia be once well developed the greatest care must be observed in the ordering of exercise. Many nervous girls have been completely broken down by following injudicious advice with regard to long walks.

THE PRINCIPLES AND PRACTICE OF MEDICINE, 1093.

474. A written list of symptoms suggests neurasthenia.

A patient with a written list of symptoms—neurasthenia.

BEAN WB. SIR WILLIAM OSLER: APHORISMS, 140.

475. One swallow does not make a summer.

Although one swallow does not make a summer, one tophus makes gout and one crescent malaria.

CUSHING H. THE LIFE OF SIR WILLIAM OSLER. VOL. 1, 594.

476. The diagnosis of a perforated appendix can be difficult.

In many instances the diagnosis of perforated appendix presents great difficulties.

TYPHLITIS AND APPENDICITIS. CAN LANCET 1888-1889;21:193-6.

477. In patients with suspected acute appendicitis, one should err toward laparotomy.

The indications for surgical interference [in cases of suspected appendicitis] are not always clear; but my experience has taught me that the abdomen is much more frequently left untouched than it should be, and that an operation is too often deferred until practically useless.

TYPHLITIS AND APPENDICITIS. CAN LANCET 1888-1889;21:193-6.

478. The pain of peptic ulcer is distinctive.

Pain is perhaps the most constant and distinctive feature of [peptic] ulcer. It varies greatly in character; it may be only a gnawing or burning sensation, which is particularly felt when the stomach is empty, and is relieved by taking food, but the more characteristic form comes on in paroxysms of the most intense gastralgia, in which the pain is not only felt in the epigastrium, but radiates to the back and to the sides.

THE PRINCIPLES AND PRACTICE OF MEDICINE, 371.

479. *The stomach is the most abused organ.*

The stomach is the hardest worked and most abused organ of the body, more subject also to irritation than any other, but it shares its unenviable position, so far as frequency of attack, with two other organs, the breast and the uterus, which live lives of comparative idleness.

CANCER OF THE STOMACH: A CLINICAL STUDY. PHILADELPHIA: P. BLAKISTON, 1900:14-5.

480. *Find romance in the abdomen.*

Area of abdominal romance—where the head of the pancreas is enfolded in the arms of the duodenum, and the liver is nestled around.

BEAN WB. SIR WILLIAM OSLER: APHORISMS, 149.

481. *The stomach is a bad neighbor to the heart.*

The stomach is not only a near but a bad neighbor to the heart.

DISEASES OF THE VALVES OF THE HEART: TREATMENT OF CARDIAC INSUFFICIENCY. IN OSLER W AND McCRAE T (EDS). MODERN MEDICINE: ITS THEORY AND PRACTICE. PHILADELPHIA: LEA & FEBIGER, 1908;4:262.

482. *Stomach troubles are due to omphalism.*

Stomach troubles are often due to omphalism of a high order—self-centered gazing at our navels.

BEAN WB. SIR WILLIAM OSLER: APHORISMS, 140.

483. *Empty the stomach.*

A greatly distended stomach is an epigastric swill barrel which should be turned up and emptied occasionally.

BEAN WB. SIR WILLIAM OSLER: APHORISMS, 147.

484. Some patients with stomach cancer lack symptoms.

One is astonished to notice how extensive and widespread the disease [cancer of the stomach] may be with practically no symptoms.

CANCER OF THE STOMACH: A CLINICAL STUDY. PHILADELPHIA: P. BLAKISTON, 1900:137.

485. Early removal of stomach cancer yields best results.

Surgical treatment—This offers the only chance of recovery. To attain the best possible results the physician and surgeon must co-operate. For the former it is the difficult question of early diagnosis, so that the cases may be placed in the hands of the surgeon at the earliest possible date.

CANCER OF THE STOMACH: A CLINICAL STUDY. PHILADELPHIA: P. BLAKISTON, 1900:152.

486. Diagnosis is often made late in the course of breast cancer.

The physician sees carcinoma of the breast at two periods. Hoping against hope, and dreading the knife, women consult him, rather than the surgeon about a "lump" which they have noticed. But far more important are the numerous and unhappy victims of the late internal metastases.

AN ADDRESS ON THE MEDICAL ASPECTS OF CARCINOMA OF THE BREAST. BRIT MED J 1906;1:1-4.

487. Symptoms may fluctuate unrelated to treatment.

We must bear in mind in these affections [leukemia and Hodgkin's disease] that there are natural periods of improvement without any special medication.

ON THE USE OF ARSENIC IN CERTAIN FORMS OF ANEMIA. THERAPEUTIC GAZ (DETROIT) 1886;2:741-6.

488. *Diagnostic accuracy is confirmed by surgery or autopsy.*

In the diagnosis of abdominal tumors Bishop Butler's [Joseph Butler (1692-1752), English philosopher and priest] maxim that "probability is the rule of life" is particularly true, and the cocksureness of the clinical physician, who formerly had to dread only the mortifying disclosures of the postmortem room, is now wisely tempered when the surgeon can so promptly and safely decide upon the nature of an obscure case.

LECTURES ON THE DIAGNOSIS OF ABDOMINAL TUMORS. NEW YORK: D. APPLETON, 1899:1-2.

489. *Bed sores recover slowly.*

Bed sores are not always a reflection on doctor or nurse...It will take as long to recover from the bed sores as from the original disease.

PRATT JH. A YEAR WITH OSLER, 24.

490. *Rapid aging is seen with progeria.*

A rare, but still more extraordinary, bodily state is that of progeria, in which, as though touched with the wand of some malign fairy, the child does not remain infantile, but skips adolescence, maturity and manhood, and passes at once to senility, looking at 11 or 12 years like a miniature Tithonus [Greek mythological hero who was granted immortality but not eternal youth. He was the subject of a poem by Tennyson (1809-1892).] "marred and wasted," wrinkled and stunted, a little old man among his toys.

VALEDICTORY ADDRESS TO THE JOHNS HOPKINS UNIVERSITY. JAMA 1905;44:705-10.

491. Post-partum hemorrhage is sometimes fatal.

The doctor may have left, feeling safe and satisfied. The attention of the nurse is attracted by a sudden restlessness of her patient, whose face shows a beginning pallor, and she finds the dressing soaked with blood. Very soon the symptoms are those of acute anemia—a rapid jerky pulse, extreme restlessness, yawning, sweating, sighing respiration, increasing pallor, and with muscular twitchings, convulsions or a sudden collapse all is over.... No wonder that novelists have made such a tragedy the climax of a story.

OBSERVATIONS ON THE SEVERE ANEMIAS OF PREGNANCY AND THE POST-PARTUM STATE.
BRIT MED J 1919;1:1-3.

492. The mentally ill have benefited from a new attitude by physicians and the public.

One of the most remarkable and beneficial reforms of the nineteenth century has been in the attitude of the profession and the public to the subject of insanity, and the gradual formation of a body of men in the profession who labour to find out the cause and means of relief of this most distressing of all human maladies.

MEDICINE IN THE NINETEENTH CENTURY, IN AEQUANIMITAS, 224.

493. The pharynx is the garbage dump.

The pharynx is the garbage dump of the bronchial tubes and nasal passages. The street sweepers (ciliated epithelial cells) are constantly on duty and especially busy at night removing the debris from the air passages to be carried away the next morning.

BEAN WB. SIR WILLIAM OSLER: APHORISMS, 134-5.

494. The triumph over juvenile hypothyroidism.

Our art has made no more brilliant advance than in the cure of these dis-orders due to disturbed function of the thyroid gland. That we can to-day rescue children otherwise doomed to helpless idiocy—that we can restore to life the hopeless victims of myxoedema—is a triumph of experimental medicine.... The results, as a rule, are most astounding—unparalleled by anything in the whole range of curative measures. Within six weeks a poor, feeble-minded, toad-like caricature of humani-ty may be restored to mental and bodily health.

THE PRINCIPLES AND PRACTICE OF MEDICINE, 3RD ED, 1898:843.

495. The hideous picture of juvenile hypothyroidism.

No type of human transformation is more distressing to look at than an aggravated case of cretinism. It recalls...those hideous transformations of the fairy prince into some frightful monster...the picture of what has been well termed the 'pariah of nature.'...Not the magic wand of Prospero [from Shakespeare's (1564-1616) The Tempest] or the brave kiss of the daughter of Hippocrates ever effected such a change as that which we are now enabled to make in these unfortunate victims, doomed heretofore to live in hopeless imbecility, an unspeakable afflic-tion to their parents and to their relatives.

SPORADIC CRETINISM IN AMERICA. TRANS CONG AM PHYS SURG 1897;4:169-206.

Lifestyle

DIET

496. Dig your grave with your teeth.

The glutton digs his own grave with his teeth.

BEAN WB. SIR WILLIAM OSLER: APHORISMS, 137.

497. We eat too much.

Lessen the intake. We all eat too much, and in no age was the saying more true that 'the platter kills more than the sword.'

AN ADDRESS ON HIGH BLOOD PRESSURE: ITS ASSOCIATIONS, ADVANTAGES, AND
DISADVANTAGES. BRIT MED J 1912;2:1173-7.

498. Eliminate careless habits of eating.

My own rule of life has been to cut out unsparingly any article of diet that had the bad taste to disagree with me, or to indicate in any way that it had abused the temporary hospitality of the lodging which I had provided.

A WAY OF LIFE, IN A WAY OF LIFE, 244-5.

499. Too much food is a health hazard.

Intemperance in the quantity of food taken is almost the rule. Adults eat far too much, and physicians are beginning to recognize that the early degenerations, particularly of the arteries and of the kidneys, leading to Bright's disease, which were formerly attributed to alcohol are due in large part to too much food.

MEDICINE IN THE NINETEENTH CENTURY, IN AEQUANIMITAS, 257.

500. Overeating is a common and important cause of disease.

People habitually eat too much, and it is probably true that a greater number of maladies arise from excess in eating than from excess in drinking.

THE PRINCIPLES AND PRACTICE OF MEDICINE, 463.

501. Eat a sensible diet.

We are all dietetic sinners; only a small percent of what we eat nourishes us, the balance goes to waste and loss of energy.

BEAN WB. SIR WILLIAM OSLER: APHORISMS, 100.

502. The importance of diet is recognized as central to health.

One of the most striking characteristics of the modern treatment of disease is the return to what used to be called the natural methods—diet, exercise, bathing and massage…. Dyspepsia, the besetting malady of this country, is largely due to improper diet, imperfectly prepared and too hastily eaten. One of the great lessons to be learned is that the preservation of health depends in great part upon food well cooked and carefully eaten. A common cause of ruined digestion, particularly in young girls, is the eating of sweets between meals and the drinking of the abominations dispensed in the chemists' shops in the form of ice-cream sodas, etc. Another frequent cause of ruined digestion in business men is the hurried meal at the lunch-counter. And a third factor, most important of all, illustrates the old maxim, that more people are killed by over eating and drinking than by the sword.

MEDICINE IN THE NINETEENTH CENTURY, IN AEQUANIMITAS, 256.

503. Obesity may have several causes.

Corpulence, an excessive development of the bodily fat—"an oily drop-sy," in the words of Lord Byron [1788-1824, English Romantic poet]—is a condition for which we are consulted in three groups of cases. First, there are persons of both sexes who have an hereditary tendency to obe-sity. Secondly, there is an increasing number of cases of obesity in chil-dren, particularly in the United States, associated with bad habits in eat-ing, and usually carelessness and lack of control on the part of the par-ents. Thirdly, and most frequently, we are consulted by women at the middle period of life, who are troubled with an over-growth of fat.... Too much food and too little exercise are largely responsible in about one half of the cases, but in the hereditary ones these factors do not pre-vail, and this is a point to be borne in mind very carefully in the ques-tion of treatment.

THE PRINCIPLES AND PRACTICE OF MEDICINE, 431.

504. Overeating after age 40 predisposes to gout.

With few exceptions, persons over forty eat too much, and the first injunction to a gouty person is to keep his appetite within reasonable bounds, to eat at stated hours, and to take plenty of time at his meals.

THE PRINCIPLES AND PRACTICE OF MEDICINE, 406.

505. We experiment with food and drink.

Disease is an experiment, and the earthly machine is a culture medium, a test tube, and a retort—the external agents, the medium and the reac-tion constituting the factors. We constantly experiment with ourselves in food and drink, and the expression so often on our lips, "Does it agree with you?" signifies how tentative are many of our daily actions.

THE EVOLUTION OF THE IDEA OF EXPERIMENT IN MEDICINE, IN TRANSACTIONS OF THE CONGRESS OF AMERICAN PHYSICIANS AND SURGEONS, SEVENTH TRIENNIAL SESSION. NEW HAVEN: BY THE CONGRESS, 1907:7.

506. How to live to a ripe old age.

Heberden's nodes, a few casts, a little albumen, mean a few clinkers—
too much stoking. We all have them after forty. Reduce meat and drink,
flush the drain pipes frequently, keep early hours, and you may yet live
to a ripe old age.

BEAN WB. SIR WILLIAM OSLER: APHORISMS, 147.

EXERCISE

507. Exercise is valuable.

Within the past quarter of a century the value of *exercise* in the education of the young has become recognized. The increase in the means of
taking wholesome out-of-door exercise is remarkable, and should show
in a few years an influence in the reduction of the nervous troubles in
young persons. The prophylactic benefit of systematic exercise, taken in
moderation by persons of middle age, is very great.

MEDICINE IN THE NINETEENTH CENTURY, IN AEQUANIMITAS, 257-8.

508. Patients need the quadrangle of health.

Patients should have rest, food, fresh air, and exercise—the quadrangle
of health.

BEAN WB. SIR WILLIAM OSLER: APHORISMS, 98.

509. Exercise is a key element in the treatment of myocardial disease.

The most important element of all [in the treatment of myocardial dis-
ease] is graduated exercise, not on the level, but on hills of various grades.
The distance walked each day is marked off and is gradually lengthened.
In this way the heart is systematically exercised and strengthened.

THE PRINCIPLES AND PRACTICE OF MEDICINE, 829.

VICES

510. *Be temperate in your vices.*

Who serves the gods die young—Venus [Greek goddess of love and beauty], Bacchus [god of wine and revelry], and Vulcan [god of fire] send in no bills in the seventh decade.

BEAN WB. SIR WILLIAM OSLER: APHORISMS, 99.

511. *Wage war against vice.*

Against our third great foe—vice in all its forms—we have to wage an incessant warfare, which is not less vigorous because of the quiet, silent kind. Better than any one else the physician can say the word in season to the immoral, to the intemperate, to the uncharitable in word and deed.

UNITY, PEACE AND CONCORD, IN AEQUANIMITAS, 437.

512. *Be temperate.*

Above all things be strictly temperate. I will not say that you are in duty bound to give up the use of stimulants altogether—though my own convictions on this point are very strong,—but this I do say, that the slightest habitual over-indulgence is as the small flaw in some dyke that forms the barrier to a mighty flood, which widening day by day, sooner or later drowns every fair promise and brings inevitable ruin.

INTRODUCTORY ADDRESS AT THE OPENING OF THE FORTY-FIFTH SESSION OF THE MEDICAL FACULTY, McGILL COLLEGE. CAN MED SURG J 1877-78;6:193-210.

513. *A drink before breakfast indicates a heavy drinker or a Southerner.*

A man who drinks before breakfast as a rule is a heavy drinker. This is not true south of Mason and Dixon's line. There a man may take his only drink before breakfast.

PRATT JH. A YEAR WITH OSLER, 3.

514. *Treatment of alcoholism is difficult.*

Chronic alcoholism is a condition very difficult to treat, and once full established the habit is rarely abandoned. The most obstinate cases are those with marked hereditary tendency.

THE PRINCIPLES AND PRACTICE OF MEDICINE, 372.

515. *Throw away the beer and spirits.*

Throw all the beer and spirits into the Irish Channel, the English Channel, and the North Sea for a year, and people in England would be infinitely better. It would certainly solve all the problems with which the philanthropists, the physicians, and the politicians have to deal.

BEAN WB. SIR WILLIAM OSLER: APHORISMS, 70.

516. *Abstinence from alcohol is the best policy.*

In every large body of men a few are to be found whose incapacity for the day results from the morning clogging of nocturnally-flushed tissues. As moderation is very hard to reach, and as it has been abundantly shown that the best of mental and physical work may be done without alcohol in any form, the safest rule for the young man is that which I am sure most of you follow—abstinence.

A WAY OF LIFE, IN AEQUANIMITAS, 245.

517. Doctors should be teetotallers.

No class of individuals can better wage war against the indiscriminate drinking habits of the public than the Doctors, and the laity will hearken to their admonitions on this point; even when the exhortations of the Divines are treated with contempt. Example, Gentlemen, is better than precept, and by becoming teetotallers yourselves, you will neither injure your health nor damage your professional prospects. Too many valuable lives in our Profession are sacrificed yearly to intemperance; and, now is the time for you, with minds still "wax to receive and marble to retain" [from *Beppo* by Lord Byron (1788-1824)] to lay the foundation of good sober habits.

VALEDICTORY ADDRESS TO THE GRADUATES IN MEDICINE AND SURGERY, McGILL
UNIVERSITY. CAN MED SURG J 1874-75;3:433-42.

518. Alcohol is a dangerous remedy.

That alcohol is a medicine, and a valuable one, nobody not blinded by prejudice denies; but bear in mind that it is a dangerous remedy, and one that should not be, as it is, so generally recommended by practitioners.

VALEDICTORY ADDRESS TO THE GRADUATES IN MEDICINE AND SURGERY, McGILL
UNIVERSITY. CAN MED SURG J 1874-75;3:433-42.

519. Prescribe alcohol with great caution.

There are many conditions, for which alcohol is now freely prescribed, quite amenable to treatment by other medicinal agents combined with a careful regulation of diet. When you do order it, give positive directions about the quantity, and the length of time it is to be continued. Inattention to these matters, especially in patients suffering from any of the neuroses, is occasionally the starting point of dangerous drinking habits.

VALEDICTORY ADDRESS TO THE GRADUATES IN MEDICINE AND SURGERY, McGILL
UNIVERSITY. CAN MED SURG J 1874-75;3:433-42.

520. Wine can be dangerous in excess.

Sensible people have begun to realize that alcoholic excesses lead invariably to impaired health...but it only too frequently happens that early in the fifth decade, just as business or political success is assured, Bacchus [Greek god of wine and revelry] hands in heavy bills for payment, in the form of serious diseases of the arteries or of the liver, or there is a general breakdown.

MEDICINE IN THE NINETEENTH CENTURY, IN AEQUANIMITAS, 256.

521. In persons with presumed acute alcoholism, consider alternative diagnoses.

The diagnosis [of acute alcoholism] is not difficult, yet mistakes are frequently made. Persons are sometimes brought to hospital by the police supposed to be drunk when in reality they are dying from apoplexy. Too great care can not be exercised, and the patient should receive the benefit of the doubt.

THE PRINCIPLES AND PRACTICE OF MEDICINE, 369.

522. Admit a dead drunk.

Alcoholism or coma? Better admit a patient to the hospital dead drunk than turn him away to be discharged from the jail dead sober a little later.

BEAN WB. SIR WILLIAM OSLER: APHORISMS, 133.

523. Tobacco affects mental clarity.

A bitter enemy to the bright eye and the clear brain of the early morning is tobacco when smoked to excess.... Watch it, test it, and if need be, control it. That befogged, woolly sensation reaching from the forehead to the occiput, that haziness of memory, that cold fish-like eye, that furred tongue, and last week's taste in the mouth—they often come from too much tobacco.

A WAY OF LIFE, IN A WAY OF LIFE, 245.

Drugs and Pharmaceutical Companies

524. It is difficult to discern prognostic factors in a disease with high mortality.

The higher the mortality the more difficult it is to estimate in any disease the value of the various elements of prognosis.

OSLER W. ON CERTAIN FEATURES IN THE PROGNOSIS OF PNEUMONIA. AM J MED SCI
1897; 113 (NEW SERIES): 1-10.

525. Correlate the autopsy with the clinical findings.

In the investigation of disease, knowledge of the morbid phenomena observed during life and the organic alterations found after death are inseparable. The teaching of the post-mortem room must supplement and illustrate the lessons of the ward.

OSLER W. NOTES ON THE MORBID ANATOMY OF PNEUMONIA. CANADA MED AND SURG
JOURNAL, 1884-1885; 13: 596-605.

526. Man's desire to take medicine is inborn.

Man has an inborn craving for medicine…the desire to take medicine is one feature which distinguishes man, the animal, from his fellow creatures.

TEACHING AND THINKING, IN AEQUANIMITAS, 125.

527. Man's capacity for self-deception with medicines is great.

The blind faith which some men have in medicines illustrates too often the greatest of all human capacities—the capacity for self-deception.

THE TREATMENT OF DISEASE. CAN LANCET 1909;42:899-912.

528. Persons with substance abuse disorders tend to lie.

Persons addicted to morphia are inveterate liars, and no reliance whatever can be placed upon their statements. In many instances this is not confined to matters relating to the vice.

THE PRINCIPLES AND PRACTICE OF MEDICINE, 374.

529. Do not be upset when your patients use alternative remedies.

"Knowledge comes, but wisdom lingers," [from "Locksley Hall" by Alfred Lord Tennyson (1809-1892)] and in matters medical the ordinary citizen of to-day has not one whit more sense than the old Romans, whom Lucian [2nd century Greek satirist] scourged for a credulity which made them fall easy victims to the quacks of the time,...Deal gently then with this deliciously credulous old human nature in which we work, and restrain your indignation, when you find your pet parson has triturates of the 1000th potentiality in his waistcoat pocket, or you discover accidentally a case of Warner's Safe Cure [a quack pill] in the bedroom of your best patient. It must needs be that offences of this kind come; expect them, and do not be vexed.

AEQUANIMITAS, IN AEQUANIMITAS, 6.

530. Our attitude towards alternative medicine should not be hostile.

I feel that our attitude as a profession should not be hostile, and we must scan gently our brother man and sister woman who may be carried away in the winds of new doctrine [alternative medicine].

THE FAITH THAT HEALS. BRIT MED J 1910;1:1470-2.

531. Cultivate a sceptical attitude toward drugs.

While on the one hand I would encourage you with the firmest faith in a few drugs ("the friends you have and their adoption tried"), on the other hand I would urge you to cultivate a keenly sceptical attitude towards the pharmacopeia as a whole, remembering the shrewd remark of Benjamin Franklin, that "he is the best doctor who knows the worthlessness of the most medicines."

THE RESERVES OF LIFE. ST. MARY'S HOSP GAZ 1907;13:95-8.

532. Do not use strange medicines.

Remember how much you do not know. Do not pour strange medicines into your patients.

THAYER, WS. OSLER THE TEACHER, IN OSLER AND OTHER PAPERS, 3.

533. Be careful with new products.

Do not rashly use every new product of which the peripatetic siren sings. Consider what surprising reactions may occur in the laboratory from the careless mixing of unknown substances.

THAYER, WS. OSLER THE TEACHER, IN OSLER AND OTHER PAPERS, 3.

534. Not every malady has a drug.

Nickel-in-the-slot, press-the-button therapeutics are no good. You cannot have a drug for every malady.

BEAN WB. SIR WILLIAM OSLER: APHORISMS, 106.

535. Avoid polypharmacy.

The battle against polypharmacy, or the use of a large number of drugs (of the action of which we know little, yet we put them into bodies of the action of which we know less), has not been fought to a finish.

MEDICINE IN THE NINETEENTH CENTURY, IN AEQUANIMITAS, 255.

536. Experienced physicians use fewer drugs.

The young physician starts life with twenty drugs for each disease, and the old physician ends life with one drug for twenty diseases.

BEAN WB. SIR WILLIAM OSLER: APHORISMS, 122.

537. Know how to use old remedies first.

In therapeutics we do not so much need new remedies as a fuller knowledge of when and how to use the old ones.

ON THE USE OF ARSENIC IN CERTAIN FORMS OF ANAEMIA. THERAPEUTICA GAZ (DETROIT) 1886;2:741-6.

538. True polypharmacy is a skillful combination.

The true polypharmacy is the skilful combination of remedies.

THE TREATMENT OF DISEASE. BRIT MED J 1909;2:185-9.

539. Too many drugs mean they are all insufficient.

If many drugs are used for a disease, all are insufficient.

BEAN WB. SIR WILLIAM OSLER: APHORISMS, 105.

540. Drugging is not the chief function of the doctor.

Imperative drugging—the ordering of medicine in any and every mala-dy—is no longer regarded as the chief function of the doctor.

MEDICINE IN THE NINETEENTH CENTURY, IN AEQUANIMITAS, 254.

541. Educate the public to avoid medicines.

One of the first duties of the physician is to educate the masses not to take medicines.

BEAN WB. SIR WILLIAM OSLER: APHORISMS, 105.

542. The commercial promotion of drugs is lamentable.

I would protest against the usurpation on the part of these men [pur-veyors of pharmaceuticals] of our function as teachers.... What right have Z. & Co. to send on a card directions for the treatment of anemia and dyspepsia, about which subjects they know as much as a newborn babe, and, if they stick to their legitimate business, about the same opportunity of getting information! For years the profession has been exploited in this way until the evil has become unbearable.

THE TREATMENT OF DISEASE. CAN LANCET 1909;42:899-912.

543. An orgy of drugging in the United States has been prolonged.

For generations the people of the United States have indulged in an orgie of drugging. Between polypharmacy in the profession, and quack medicines, the American body had become saturated *ad nauseum*.

THE FAITH THAT HEALS. BRIT MED J 1910;1:1470-2.

544. Treatment is controlled by pharmaceutical manufacturers.

Far too large a section of the treatment of disease is to-day controlled by the big manufacturing pharmacists, who have enslaved us in a plausible pseudo-science. The remedy is obvious—give our students a first-hand acquaintance with disease and give them a thorough practical knowledge of the great drugs and we will send out independent, clear-headed, cautious practitioners who will do their own thinking and be no longer at the mercy of a meretricious literature which has sapped our independence.

THE TREATMENT OF DISEASE. CAN LANCET 1909;42:899-912.

6

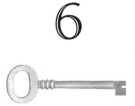

Medical Education

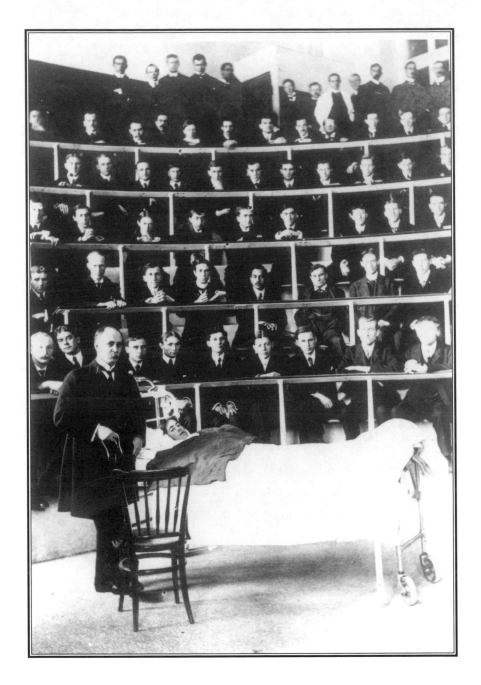

William Osler conducting a clinic while visiting
Royal Victoria Hospital, McGill University, in 1906.
(Courtesy of Richard L. Golden, MD.)

Medical Education

The Medical Student

545. *Learn to recognize and to treat disease.*

You may as students haste to rise up early and late take rest; you may eat the bread of carefulness and it will be but lost labor if you have not, when you go among your fellow men, the practical information needful for the successful recognition and treatment of disease. As I said at the onset you are gathered here for this purpose and should have no other object, no other ambition.

UNPUBLISHED DRAFT OF AN ADDRESS TO MEDICAL STUDENTS AT THE UNIVERSITY OF PENNSYLVANIA, 1885. PUBLISHED PRIVATELY BY THE OSLER LIBRARY, McGILL UNIVERSITY, MONTREAL, 2006.

546. The student must observe the patient as carefully as if he was in charge.

Under a proper system, he must see that patient from day to day, note the progress, the various phases of the disease, the complications that arise and the action of the medicines. He must watch that case as a student just as carefully as if he was in practice and had sole charge of it. This is clinical medicine.

UNPUBLISHED DRAFT OF AN ADDRESS TO MEDICAL STUDENTS AT THE UNIVERSITY OF

PENNSYLVANIA, 1885. PUBLISHED PRIVATELY BY THE OSLER LIBRARY, MCGILL

UNIVERSITY, MONTREAL, 2006.

547. The student must learn to collect, record, compare, reason, and prescribe.

The student and the patient must stand in the same relation as the anatomist and his subject, the chemist and his solution. He must be put in a position to get for himself, under supervision, the facts relating to the patient's malady, which he must collect, record and compare; he must be taught to reason correctly upon them, to weigh the evidence in any given case and then prescribe the appropriate remedies.

UNPUBLISHED DRAFT OF AN ADDRESS TO MEDICAL STUDENTS AT THE UNIVERSITY OF

PENNSYLVANIA, 1885. PUBLISHED PRIVATELY BY THE OSLER LIBRARY, MCGILL

UNIVERSITY, MONTREAL, 2006.

548. The physician is called to combat disease.

Whereas the Biologist studies his objects with the sole purpose of gaining information upon their life and processes, the Physician looks further to the great object of his calling, the accurate knowledge of the modes of combating those phenomena which we call abnormal or diseased.

UNPUBLISHED DRAFT OF AN ADDRESS TO MEDICAL STUDENTS AT THE UNIVERSITY OF

PENNSYLVANIA, 1885. PUBLISHED PRIVATELY BY THE OSLER LIBRARY, MCGILL

UNIVERSITY, MONTREAL, 2006.

549. Basic science is essential to clinical medicine.

When a student knows the structure of the body and the functions of the various organs [and] the chemistry of the secretions in health and the properties and composition of drugs, there and then only is he ready to enter upon the study of his profession.

UNPUBLISHED DRAFT OF AN ADDRESS TO MEDICAL STUDENTS AT THE UNIVERSITY OF PENNSYLVANIA, 1885. PUBLISHED PRIVATELY BY THE OSLER LIBRARY, MCGILL UNIVERSITY, MONTREAL, 2006.

550. True progress is slow.

Practical anatomy develops qualities in the student which stand by him in every subsequent position. He is taught at once the lesson, so hard to learn, that all true progress is slow and by successive steps.

UNPUBLISHED DRAFT OF AN ADDRESS TO MEDICAL STUDENTS AT THE UNIVERSITY OF PENNSYLVANIA, 1885. PUBLISHED PRIVATELY BY THE OSLER LIBRARY, MCGILL UNIVERSITY, MONTREAL, 2006.

551. The student is an object of study.

Except it be a lover, no one is more interesting as an object of study than a student. Shakespeare [1564-1616] might have made him a fourth in his immortal group. The lunatic with his fixed idea, the poet with his fine frenzy, the lover with his frantic idolatry, and the student aflame with the desire for knowledge are of "imagination all compact." [from *A Midsummer Night's Dream*]

THE STUDENT LIFE, IN AEQUANIMITAS, 397.

552. *Accept the limitations of humans.*

What is the student but a lover courting a fickle mistress who ever eludes his grasp? In this very elusiveness is brought out his second great characteristic—steadfastness of purpose. Unless from the start the limitations incident to our frail human faculties are frankly accepted, nothing but disappointment awaits you.

THE STUDENT LIFE, IN AEQUANIMITAS, 398.

553. *A student should be a citizen of the world.*

The true student is a citizen of the world, the allegiance of whose soul, at any rate, is too precious to be restricted to a single country. The great minds, the great works transcend all limitations of time, of language, and of race, and the scholar can never feel initiated into the company of the elect until he can approach all of life's problems from the cosmopolitan viewpoint. I care not in what subject he may work, the full knowledge cannot be reached without drawing on supplies from other lands than his own—French, English, German, American, Japanese, Russian, Italian—there must be no discrimination by the loyal student, who should willingly draw from any and every source with an open mind and a stern resolve to render unto all their dues.

THE STUDENT LIFE, IN AEQUANIMITAS, 401.

554. *The qualities of a true student are easily recognized.*

The [true student] defies definition, but there are three unmistakable signs by which you can recognize the genuine article...an absorbing desire to know the truth, an unswerving steadfastness in its pursuit, and an open, honest heart, free from suspicion, guile, and jealousy.

THE STUDENT LIFE, IN A WAY OF LIFE, 171.

555. A genius is one who does it easily.

You can all become good students, a few may become great students, and now and again one of you will be found who does easily and well what others cannot do at all, or very badly, which is John Ferriar's [(1764-1815), Scottish physician, reformer, essayist, and poet] excellent definition of a genius.

THE STUDENT LIFE, IN A WAY OF LIFE, 174.

556. Medical students will do well.

I never met a crowd of medical students but I think of [John] Abernethy's [(1764-1831), British surgeon and founder of St. Bartholomew's Hospital Medical School in London] remark, "Good God! What will become of you all." I know what will become of you. You will all do well.

DR. OSLER TO STUDENTS. OKLAHOMA MED J 1900;8:53.

557. Never lose sight of your goal.

Never lose sight of the end and object of all your studies; the cure of disease and the alleviation of suffering. Some of you will soon be placed in the chamber of the sick, by the bed-side of the dying, and the issues of life and death may be in your hands. Think of this now, and while you have time use your talents aright. Your lives will be a constant warfare against a common enemy, implacable, often irresistible, who spares neither age nor sex, and who, too often, as the memories of the past week remind us, turns and bitterly avenges the victories of those who have many a time snatched victims from his grasp.

INTRODUCTORY LECTURE, 18.

558. Your mission is to fight disease and death.

So it will be your highest mission, students of medicine, to carry on the never-ending warfare against disease and death, better equipped, abler men than your predecessors, but animated with their spirit, and sustained by their hopes "for the hope of every creature is the banner that we bear."

TEACHING AND THINKING, IN AEQUANIMITAS, 126.

559. Education is a life course.

The hardest conviction to get into the mind of a beginner is that the education upon which he is engaged is not a college course, not a medical course, but a life course, for which the work of a few years under teachers is but a preparation.

THE STUDENT LIFE, IN AEQUANIMITAS, 400.

560. Learning is lifelong.

At the outset it is necessary for you to bear in mind that your professional education [on graduation] is by no means complete; you have, as it were, only laid the foundation, and,...while it is to be hoped that a good and promising foundation has been laid under the guidance and instruction of others, it rests with yourselves what the superstructure shall be.

VALEDICTORY ADDRESS TO THE GRADUATES IN MEDICINE AND SURGERY, MCGILL COLLEGE. CAN MED SURG J 1874-75;3:433-42.

561. Medicine is a difficult art to acquire.

Medicine is a most difficult art to acquire. All the college can do is to teach the student principles, based on facts in science, and give him good methods of work. These simply start him in the right direction, they do not make a good practitioner—that is his own affair. To master the art requires sustained effort, like the bird's flight which depends on the incessant action of the wings, but this sustained effort is so hard that many give up the struggle in despair.

MEDICINE AND NURSING. IN MATHEWS B (ED). ESSAYS ON VOCATION. LONDON:

OXFORD UNIVERSITY PRESS, 1919:7.

562. The practical outcome of medical training is to help others.

For consider the practical outcome of all the knowledge you gather; the active work for which your four years' study is a preparation. Will not your whole energies be spent in befriending the sick and suffering? in helping those who cannot help themselves? in rescuing valuable lives from the clutch of grim disease? in cheering the loving nurses of the sick, who often hang upon your words with a most touching trust?

INTRODUCTORY LECTURE, 5.

563. The path of medical education follows the evolution of knowledge.

Just as the embryo passes through life of lower grade, before resulting in the thinking man—the ontogeny reproducing the phylogeny—so the career of the medical student follows the evolution of the marvellous knowledge that has made our profession the most helpful of all to humanity.

THE PATHOLOGICAL INSTITUTE OF A GENERAL HOSPITAL. GLASGOW MED J

1911;76:321-33.

564. Medicine is progressive.

The credit of your College, the honour of that Profession, to which it is our privilege and pleasure to belong, your advancement in life depend on the course you now mark out and follow for yourselves. You must not be content to rest on your oars. The canons of the church, the formulas of the law, are to a certain extent unalterable, are stereotyped. Not so medicine. It is pre-eminently a progressive science, day by day receiving fresh acquisitions, opening up new fields for investigation, and it will be your duty, as far as in you lies, to keep pace with this progress.

VALEDICTORY ADDRESS TO THE GRADUATES IN MEDICINE AND SURGERY, MCGILL COLLEGE. CAN MED SURG J 1874-75;3:433-42.

565. Medical school only gives direction.

The training of the medical school gives a man his direction, points him the way, and furnishes him with a chart, fairly incomplete, for the voyage, but nothing more.

BEAN WB. SIR WILLIAM OSLER: APHORISMS, 40.

566. It is not an advantage to begin clinical work early.

Much as I love hospital work and much as I believe in the life of the student in the hospital, I do not think that, with our present congested curriculum, it is an advantage to begin clinical work at once. It may be good for the medical student morally, but I am sure it is bad for him intellectually, and he gleans a heterogeneous accumulation of isolated half-understood experiences, instead of an orderly sequence, in which the acquired knowledge of laboratories is brought to bear on the problems of disease.

IMPRESSIONS OF PARIS. I. TEACHERS AND STUDENTS. JAMA 1909;52:771-4.

567. Students should divide their attentions between books and patients.

Divide your attentions equally between books and men. The strength of the student of books is to sit still—two or three hours at a stretch—eating the heart out of a subject with pencil and notebook in hand, determined to master the details and intricacies, focussing all your energies on its difficulties. Get accustomed to test all sorts of book problems and statements for yourself, and take as little as possible on trust.

THE STUDENT LIFE, IN AEQUANIMITAS, 405.

568. Students learn to study disease and treat patients.

The pupil handles a sufficient number of cases to get a certain measure of technical skill, and there is ever kept before him the idea that he is not in the hospital to learn everything that is known but to learn how to study disease and how to treat it, or rather, as I prefer to teach, how to treat patients.

ON THE NEED OF A RADICAL REFORM IN OUR METHODS OF TEACHING SENIOR STUDENTS. MED NEWS [NEW YORK] 1903;82:49-53.

569. The disease should be the teacher.

He does not see the pneumonia case in the amphitheatre from the benches, but he follows it day by day, hour by hour; he has his time so arranged that he can follow it; he sees and studies similar cases and the disease itself becomes his chief teacher, and he knows its phases and variations as depicted in the living; he learns under skilled direction when to act and when to refrain, he learns insensibly principles of practice and he possibly escapes a "nickel-in-the-slot" attitude of mind which has been the curse of the physician in the treatment of disease.

THE FIXED PERIOD, IN AEQUANIMITAS, 389.

570. Put the student in the wards.

How can we make the work of the student in the third and fourth year as practical as it is in his first and second?…The answer is, take him from the lecture-room, take him from the amphitheatre,—put him in the out-patient department—put him in the wards.

ON THE NEED FOR A RADICAL REFORM IN OUR METHODS OF TEACHING SENIOR STUDENTS. MED NEWS [NEW YORK] 1903;82:49-53.

571. *In teaching, emphasize methods, not facts.*

We expect too much of the student and we try to teach him too much. Give him good methods and a proper point of view, and all other things will be added, as his experience grows.

ON THE NEED OF A RADICAL REFORM IN OUR METHODS OF TEACHING SENIOR STUDENTS. MED NEWS [NEW YORK] 1903;82:49-53.

572. *We try to teach too much.*

Undoubtedly the student tries to learn too much, and we teachers try to teach him too much—neither, perhaps, with great success.

AFTER TWENTY-FIVE YEARS, IN AEQUANIMITAS, 201.

573. *Reform the curriculum.*

The student needs more time for quiet study, fewer classes, fewer lectures, and, above all, the incubus of examinations should be lifted from his soul. To replace the Chinese by the Greek spirit would enable him to seek knowledge for itself, without a thought of the end, tested and taught day by day, the pupil and teacher working together on the same lines, only one a little ahead of the other. This is the ideal towards which we should move.

AN INTRODUCTORY ADDRESS ON EXAMINATIONS, EXAMINERS, AND EXAMINEES. LANCET 1913;2:1047-50.

574. *Medical students need to learn how to become practical physicians.*

Every medical student should remember that his end is not to be made a chemist or physiologist or anatomist, but to learn how to recognize and treat disease, how to become a practical physician.

AFTER TWENTY-FIVE YEARS, IN AEQUANIMITAS, 205.

575. What the medical student should learn in the hospital is limited.

The stay of the medical student in the hospital is so brief, the amount to be learned so vast, that we can only hope to give him two things—method (technique) and such elementary knowledge as how to examine patients, the life history of a few great diseases and the great principles of surgical practice.

SPECIALISM IN THE GENERAL HOSPITAL. JOHNS HOPKINS HOSP BULL 1913;24:167-71.

576. Time is too short to learn both general medicine and the specialties.

The art is getting longer and longer, the brain of the medical student, not getting bigger and bigger, has its limits; and though keener and more industrious than ever in history, the time is too short for a man already burdened to the breaking point, to study any specialty from the standpoint of the specialist.

SPECIALISM IN THE GENERAL HOSPITAL. JOHNS HOPKINS HOSP BULL 1913;24:167-71.

577. The value of the medical student to the hospital is under-appreciated.

That the medical student is an essential factor in the life of a great general hospital, has been of slow recognition in this country.

SPECIALISM IN THE GENERAL HOSPITAL. JOHNS HOPKINS HOSP BULL 1913;24:167-71.

578. Come to your teachers for advice.

You come now into the society not of mere professors, who will lecture at you from a distance, but of men who are anxious for your welfare, who will sympathize with your difficulties and also bear with your weakness.... Look upon us as elder brothers to whom you can come confidently and fearlessly for advice in any trouble or difficulty.

PRATT JH. OSLER AS HIS STUDENTS KNEW HIM. BOSTON MED SURG J 1920;
182:338-41.

579. *Assume responsibility for your actions.*

No longer subject to the narrow rules of school-boy days and to the penalties that enforce them; released from the gentler, but no less real, restraints of home; bound only by the laws of his Alma Mater, which demand little from him that he would not willingly give, the youth feels himself for the first time his own master, and the sense of freedom rouses the growing manhood within him and gives impulse to that self-reliance and independence of action that in after years brace the man for the deeper responsibilities of life, when the power to choose is no longer a delightful novelty, but an anxious care.

INTRODUCTORY LECTURE, 15-6.

580. *The fear of failure underlies every effort.*

The fear of failure underlies every effort, and this fear must be specially present to those who run the competitive race of a university career, in which a man naturally desires, not only to reach the standard which shall secure him his degree, but also to take a high place among his fellows. This fear of failure abides with some, paralyzing their energies and growing more burdensome as time wears on and their test day is near. But let the student take courage; for though in the nature of things only one man can carry off the highest honours, I doubt if there be one among you who cannot come out well at the end of the session if he will only work as he ought.

INTRODUCTORY LECTURE, 16.

581. *Make your parents proud.*

Like some soft, familiar melody running through the clangour of martial music, the thought of home must needs mingle with all others, till
the student's fondest hope is the hope that he may be the pride of those
who have cherished him from his childhood; his firmest resolve the
resolve to do nothing unworthy of their trust in him; his holiest ambition to satisfy their loving desires for his welfare and advancement.

INTRODUCTORY LECTURE, 15.

582. *Enjoy the student life.*

Learn to love the freedom of the student life, only too quickly to pass
away; the absence of the coarser cares of after days, the joy in comradeship, the delight in new work, the happiness in knowing that you are
making progress. Once only can you enjoy these pleasures.

THE MASTER-WORD IN MEDICINE, IN AEQUANIMITAS, 362.

583. *Straddle a hobby and ride it hard.*

The young doctor should look about early for an avocation, a pastime,
that will take him away from patients, pills and potions…. No man is
really happy or safe without one, and it makes precious little difference
what the outside interest may be—botany, beetles or butterflies, roses,
tulips or irises, fishing, mountaineering or antiquities—anything will do
so long as he straddles a hobby and rides it hard.

THE MEDICAL LIBRARY IN POST-GRADUATE WORK. BRIT MED J 1909;2:925-8.

584. *Maintain outside interests.*

Get early this relish, this clear, keen joyance in work, with which languor
disappears and all shadows of annoyance flee away. But do not get too
deeply absorbed [in your work] to the exclusion of all outside interests.

Success in life depends as much upon the man as on the physician. Mix with your fellow students, mingle with their sports and their pleasures.... You are to be members of a polite as well as of a liberal profession and the more you see of life outside the narrow circle of your work the better equipped will you be for the struggle.

AFTER TWENTY-FIVE YEARS, IN AEQUANIMITAS, 203-4.

585. Seek new environments and become independent.

It is more particularly on the younger men that I would urge the advantages of an early devotion to a peripatetic philosophy of life. Just so soon as you have your second teeth think of a change; get away from the nurse, cut the apron strings of your old teachers, seek new ties in a fresh environment, if possible, where you can have a certain measure of freedom and independence.

VALEDICTORY ADDRESS TO THE JOHNS HOPKINS UNIVERSITY. JAMA 1905;44:705-10.

586. Emancipate the student.

Let us emancipate the student, and give him time and opportunity for the cultivation of his mind, so that in his pupilage he shall not be a puppet in the hands of others, but rather a self-relying and reflecting being.

BEAN WB. SIR WILLIAM OSLER: APHORISMS, 44.

587. Acquire the three reserves for the long race of medical life.

How may you acquire these reserves? The few who reached Charing Cross [a street in London] did so because of three factors: you were built for the race-track, you were properly trained, and you knew the road; and for the long race ahead these same three factors are the essentials.

THE RESERVES OF LIFE. ST. MARY'S HOSP GAZ 1907;13:95-8.

588. Take care of your body.

Some of us are congenitally unhappy during the early hours; but the young man who feels on awakening that life is a burden or a bore has been neglecting his machine, driving it too hard, stoking the engines too much, or not cleaning out the ashes and clinkers. Or he has been too much with the Lady Nicotine, or fooling with Bacchus [god of wine and revelry], or, worst of all, with the younger Aphrodite [goddess of love and beauty]— all 'messengers of strong prevailment in unhardened youth.'

A WAY OF LIFE, IN A WAY OF LIFE, 244.

589. Avoid temptations.

And now, remembering that we have other duties towards you than teaching the details of your profession, I would on this occasion earnestly impress upon you the necessity of living upright, honest, and sober lives. The way of the medical student is beset with many temptations, and too often the track he leaves is marked by as many lapses; a zig-zag path, "to right or left, eternal swervin'."

INTRODUCTORY ADDRESS AT THE OPENING OF THE FORTY-FIFTH SESSION OF THE MEDICAL FACULTY, MCGILL COLLEGE. CAN MED SURG J 1877-78;6:193-210.

590. Moral death is a tragedy.

To the teacher-nurse it is a sore disappointment to find at the end of ten years so few minds with the full stature, of which the early days gave promise. Still, so widespread is mental death that we scarcely comment upon it in our friends. The real tragedy is the moral death which, in different forms, overtakes so many good fellows who fall away from the pure, honourable, and righteous service of Minerva [goddess of wisdom, skill and invention] into the idolatry of Bacchus [god of wine and revelry], of Venus [goddess of love and beauty], or of Circe [an enchantress who turned men into swine].

THE STUDENT LIFE, IN AEQUANIMITAS, 422.

591. *Remember the loss of promising minds.*

Let us sometimes think of those who have fallen in the battle of life, who have striven and failed, who have failed even without the strife. How many have I lost from the student band by mental death, and from so many causes—some stillborn from college, others dead within the first year of infantile marasmus, while mental rickets, teething, tabes, and fits have carried off many of the most promising minds!

THE STUDENT LIFE, IN AEQUANIMITAS, 422.

592. *The loss of former students is poignant.*

Less painful to dwell upon, though associated with a more poignant grief, is the fate of those whom physical death has snatched away in the bud or blossom of the student life. These are among the tender memories of the teacher's life, of which he does not often care to speak, feeling with Longfellow that the surest pledge of their remembrance is "the silent homage of thoughts unspoken." [from "The Herons of Elmwood" by Henry Wadsworth Longfellow (1824-1884)]

THE STUDENT LIFE, IN AEQUANIMITAS, 422.

593. *The teacher (Osler) still has a lot to learn.*

It is a good many years since I sat on the benches, but I am happy to say that I am still a medical student, and still feel that I have much to learn.

ADDRESS TO THE STUDENTS OF THE ALBANY MEDICAL COLLEGE. ALBANY MED ANN
1899;20:307-9.

594. *The start of a career is heart-stirring.*

To a man who has made his start in life, who having chosen his path is now following it day by day, there is something heart-stirring in the sight of a number of young men ... just entering on the race which they will run with such varied powers, with such different results, in the busy arena of the world. For he knows that on such an occasion their hearts must be seething with thoughts of the future and of all that it may be to them. What high hopes swell the breasts before him! What earnest resolves are hidden behind the brave young faces! What steadfast aims are set as the goal which shall reward the worker for each "passionate bright endeavour" that he makes! Surely such thoughts are to each man among you as a trumpet-call, summoning the young recruit to fall into his rank on the battlefield of life.

INTRODUCTORY LECTURE, 15.

595. The opportunities are still great in internal medicine.

I have heard the fear expressed that in this country the sphere of the physician proper is becoming more and more restricted, and perhaps this is true; but I maintain (and I hope to convince you) that the opportunities are still great, that the harvest truly is plenteous, and the labourers scarcely sufficient to meet the demand.

INTERNAL MEDICINE AS A VOCATION, IN AEQUANIMITAS, 133.

596. The public should endow medical schools and hospitals.

The whole question of the practical education of the medical student is one in which the public is vitally interested. Sane, intelligent physicians and surgeons with culture, science and art are worth much in a community, and they are worth paying for in rich endowments of our medical schools and hospitals.

VALEDICTORY ADDRESS TO THE JOHNS HOPKINS UNIVERSITY. JAMA 1905;44:705-10.

Education

597. *Following a patient outmatches many lectures.*

One or two such cases followed by the student in detail are worth a dozen lectures.

UNPUBLISHED DRAFT OF AN ADDRESS TO MEDICAL STUDENTS AT THE UNIVERSITY OF
PENNSYLVANIA, 1885. PUBLISHED PRIVATELY BY THE OSLER LIBRARY, MCGILL
UNIVERSITY, MONTREAL, 2006.

598. *Lectures are not enough preparation.*

The clinical lecture has important uses too, but you cannot prepare yourselves for the work of life by sitting on the benches, no matter how interesting and varied the cases or how instructive the Professor.

UNPUBLISHED DRAFT OF AN ADDRESS TO MEDICAL STUDENTS AT THE UNIVERSITY OF
PENNSYLVANIA, 1885. PUBLISHED PRIVATELY BY THE OSLER LIBRARY, MCGILL
UNIVERSITY, MONTREAL, 2006.

599. *Avoid the pitfall of hasty inference.*

This is really one of the most serious difficulties which students have to overcome in clinical work – hasty inference from imperfectly or even well observed facts.

UNPUBLISHED DRAFT OF AN ADDRESS TO MEDICAL STUDENTS AT THE UNIVERSITY OF
PENNSYLVANIA, 1885. PUBLISHED PRIVATELY BY THE OSLER LIBRARY, MCGILL
UNIVERSITY, MONTREAL, 2006.

600. *Scientific education facilitates clinical work.*

The facility with which you will undertake clinical work depends entirely upon the thoroughness of your education in scientific branches. Well for you if you bring a knowledge which is practical, senses which have been trained to exact observation, habits painstaking and careful and above all an appreciation of the value of method in work. Thus equipped the labor will be easy and your progress rapid.

UNPUBLISHED DRAFT OF AN ADDRESS TO MEDICAL STUDENTS AT THE UNIVERSITY OF PENNSYLVANIA, 1885. PUBLISHED PRIVATELY BY THE OSLER LIBRARY, MCGILL UNIVERSITY, MONTREAL, 2006.

601. Facts alone are not enough.

Facts alone will not be of much service to you unless studied in connection with others and with the phenomena displayed during life.

UNPUBLISHED DRAFT OF AN ADDRESS TO MEDICAL STUDENTS AT THE UNIVERSITY OF PENNSYLVANIA, 1885. PUBLISHED PRIVATELY BY THE OSLER LIBRARY, MCGILL UNIVERSITY, MONTREAL, 2006.

602. The hospital is an experimental laboratory to study patients.

You will do well to regard the Hospital as a laboratory in which the patients represent so many experiments of nature which you must study and observe in a manner very similar to that which you have followed in Biology and Chemistry.

UNPUBLISHED DRAFT OF AN ADDRESS TO MEDICAL STUDENTS AT THE UNIVERSITY OF PENNSYLVANIA, 1885. PUBLISHED PRIVATELY BY THE OSLER LIBRARY, MCGILL UNIVERSITY, MONTREAL, 2006.

603. Physiology is anatomy enlightened.

Beautiful and enticing as is the study of Anatomy we cannot see its full beauty until in Physiology we study the relations of function to structure. It is a pity that the enormous development of the latter subject, Physiology, has necessitated a divorce in the teaching of what practically constitutes one science. What does it mean? Physiology is only Anatomy enlightened.

UNPUBLISHED DRAFT OF AN ADDRESS TO MEDICAL STUDENTS AT THE UNIVERSITY OF PENNSYLVANIA, 1885.PUBLISHED PRIVATELY BY THE OSLER LIBRARY, McGILL UNIVERSITY, MONTREAL, 2006.

604. Knowledge promotes love.

True and great love springs out of great knowledge, and where you know little you can love but little or not at all.

BARKER LF. DR. OSLER AS THE YOUNG PHYSICIAN'S FRIEND AND EXEMPLAR. IN ABBOTT ME (ED). SIR WILLIAM OSLER MEMORIAL NUMBER. BULLETIN NO. IX OF THE INTERNATIONAL ASSOCIATION OF MEDICAL MUSEUMS AND JOURNAL OF TECHNICAL METHODS. MONTREAL: PRIVATELY PRINTED, 1926:257.

605. Practical knowledge is real knowledge.

The knowledge which a man can use is the only real knowledge, the only knowledge which has life and growth in it and converts itself into practical power. The rest hangs like dust around the brain or dries like raindrops off stones.

FINNEY JMT. A PERSONAL APPRECIATION OF SIR WILLIAM OSLER. IN ABBOTT ME (ED). SIR WILLIAM OSLER MEMORIAL NUMBER. BULLETIN NO. IX OF THE INTERNATIONAL ASSOCIATION OF MEDICAL MUSEUMS AND JOURNAL OF TECHNICAL METHODS. MONTREAL: PRIVATELY PRINTED, 1926:281.

606. Converting knowledge into practical wisdom is difficult.

That was a very happy remark of Alfred Lord Tennyson [(1809-1892), Poet Laureate of England], 'knowledge grows but wisdom lingers.' After all, the greatest difficulty of life is to make knowledge effective, to convert it into practical wisdom. We often confuse the two, thinking they are identical. But it was another poet—Cowper [William Cowper (1731-1800), English poet]—who said that far from being one they often have no connection whatever. Now, wisdom is simply knowledge made efficient.

WHAT THE PUBLIC CAN DO IN THE FIGHT AGAINST TUBERCULOSIS. OXFORD: HORACE HART, 1909, 1-7.

607. The mind is the measure of a nation.

We forget that the measure of the value of a nation to the world is neither the bushel nor the barrel, but *mind;* and that wheat and pork, though useful and necessary, are but dross in comparison with those intellectual products which alone are imperishable. The kindly fruits of the earth are easily grown; the finer fruits of the mind are of slower development and require prolonged culture.

TEACHER AND STUDENT, IN AEQUANIMITAS, 28-9.

608. Few minds attain maturity.

It takes great care on the part of any one to live a mental life corresponding to the ages or phases through which his body passes. How few minds reach puberty, how few come to adolescence, how few attain maturity! It is really tragic—this widespread prevalence of mental infantilism, due to careless habits of intellectual feedings.

VALEDICTORY ADDRESS TO THE JOHNS HOPKINS UNIVERSITY. JAMA 1905;44:705-10.

609. Gain wisdom by collecting and using data.

What we call sense or wisdom is knowledge, ready for use, made effective, and bears the same relation to knowledge itself that bread does to wheat. The full knowledge of the parts of a steam engine and the theory of its action may be possessed by a man who could not be trusted to pull the lever to its throttle. It is only by collecting data and using them that you can get sense.

THE STUDENT LIFE, IN AEQUANIMITAS, 413.

610. Disperse ignorance.

Full knowledge, which alone disperses the mists of ignorance, can only be obtained by travel or by a thorough acquaintance with the literature of the different countries.

CHAUVINISM IN MEDICINE, IN AEQUANIMITAS, 272.

611. Learn medicine at the bedside.

Medicine is learned by the bedside and not in the classroom. Let not your conceptions of the manifestations of disease come from words heard in the lecture room or read from the book. See, and then reason and compare and control. But see first. No two eyes see the same thing. No two mirrors give forth the same reflection.... Live in the ward.

THAYER WS. OSLER THE TEACHER, IN OSLER AND OTHER PAPERS, 1.

612. Seeing is not knowing.

It is a common error to think that the more a doctor sees the greater his experience and the more he knows.

THE STUDENT LIFE, IN AEQUANIMITAS, 412.

613. The value of experience is to see wisely.

The important thing is to make the lesson of each case tell on your education. The value of experience is not in seeing much, but in seeing wisely. Experience in the true sense of the term does not come to all with years, or with increasing opportunities. Growth in the acquisition of facts is not necessarily associated with development. Many grow through life mentally as the crystal, by simple accretion, and at fifty possess, to vary the figure, the unicellular mental blastoderm with which they started.

THE ARMY SURGEON, IN AEQUANIMITAS, 105.

614. Wisdom comes from relating facts and experience.

The facts are looked at in connexion with similar ones, their relation to others is studied, and the experience of the recorder is compared with that of others who have worked upon the question. Insensibly, year by year, a man finds that there has been in his mental protoplasm not only growth by assimilation but an actual development, bringing fuller powers of observation, additional capabilities of mental nutrition, and that increased breadth of view which is of the very essence of wisdom.

THE ARMY SURGEON, IN AEQUANIMITAS, 105-6.

615. Each case has a lesson.

Each case has its lesson—a lesson that may be, but is not always, learnt, for clinical wisdom is not the equivalent of experience. A man who has seen 500 cases of pneumonia may not have the understanding of the disease which comes with an intelligent study of a score of cases, so different are knowledge and wisdom, which, as the poet truly says, "far from being one have oft-times no connexion."

ON THE EDUCATIONAL VALUE OF THE MEDICAL SOCIETY, IN AEQUANIMITAS, 335.

616. Learn from each patient.

Faithfulness in the day of small things will insensibly widen your powers, correct your faculties, and, in moments of despondency, comfort may be derived from a knowledge that some of the best work of the profession has come from men whose clinical work was limited but well-tilled. The important thing is to make the lesson of each case tell on your education.

THE ARMY SURGEON, IN AEQUANIMITAS, 105.

617. Cases are stepping-stones to clinical development.

Look at the cases not from the standpoint of text-books and monographs, but as so many stepping-stones in the progress of your individual development in the art.

THE ARMY SURGEON, IN AEQUANIMITAS, 104.

618. Every patient is a lesson.

Every patient you see is a lesson in much more than the malady from which he suffers.

THE STUDENT LIFE, IN AEQUANIMITAS, 406.

619. Learn from your errors.

Start out with the conviction that absolute truth is hard to reach in matters relating to our fellow creatures, healthy or diseased, that slips in observation are inevitable even with the best trained faculties, that errors in judgment must occur in the practice of an art which consists largely of balancing probabilities;—start, I say, with this attitude in mind, and mistakes will be acknowledged and regretted; but instead of a slow process of self-deception, with ever increasing inability to recognize truth, you will draw from your errors the very lessons which may enable you to avoid their repetition.

TEACHER AND STUDENT, IN AEQUANIMITAS, 38.

620. Learn from your mistakes.

It is always better to do a thing wrong the first time.

PENFIELD W. A MEDICAL STUDENT'S MEMORIES OF THE REGIUS PROFESSOR. IN ABBOTT ME (ED). SIR WILLIAM OSLER MEMORIAL NUMBER. BULLETIN NO. IX OF THE

INTERNATIONAL ASSOCIATION OF MEDICAL MUSEUMS AND JOURNAL OF TECHNICAL METHODS. MONTREAL: PRIVATELY PRINTED, 1926:386.

621. Let nothing slip by.

Let nothing slip by you; the ordinary humdrum cases of the morning routine may have been accurately described and pictured, but study each one separately as though it were new—so it is so far as your special experience goes; and if the spirit of the student is in you the lesson will be there.

THE ARMY SURGEON, IN AEQUANIMITAS, 104.

622. Teach students to observe the facts.

The student starts...as an observer of disordered machines, with the structure and orderly functions of which he is perfectly familiar. Teach him how to observe, give him plenty of facts to observe and the lessons will come out of the facts themselves.

ON THE NEED OF A RADICAL REFORM IN OUR METHODS OF TEACHING SENIOR STUDENTS. MED NEWS [NEW YORK] 1903;82:49-53.

623. How to acquire clinical wisdom.

It is only by persistent intelligent study of disease upon a methodical plan of examination that a man gradually learns to correlate his daily lessons with the facts of his previous experience and of that of his fellows, and so acquires clinical wisdom.

CHAUVINISM IN MEDICINE, IN AEQUANIMITAS, 282.

624. Medicine learned at the bedside is different from that in school.

Ask any physician of 20 years' standing how he has become proficient in his art, and he will reply, by constant contact with disease; and he will add that the medicine he learned in the school was totally different from the medicine he learned at the bedside.

ON THE NEED OF A RADICAL REFORM IN OUR METHODS OF TEACHING SENIOR
STUDENTS. MED NEWS [NEW YORK] 1903;82:49-53.

625. Education should prepare.

To be of any value an education should prepare for life's work.

AN INTRODUCTORY ADDRESS ON EXAMINATIONS, EXAMINERS, AND EXAMINEES. LANCET
1913;2:1047-50.

626. Appreciate the aims of medical education.

At the outset appreciate clearly the aims and objects each one of you should have in view—a knowledge of disease and its cure, and a knowledge of yourself. The one, special education, will make you a practitioner of medicine; the other, an inner education, may make you a truly good man, four square and without a flaw.

THE MASTER-WORD IN MEDICINE, IN AEQUANIMITAS, 358.

627. Society is built upon a tripod of education, health care, and law enforcement.

The conglomeration which we call society is built upon a tripod—the school-house, the hospital and the jail, which minister respectively to the manners, the maladies and the morals of man.

ON THE INFLUENCE OF A HOSPITAL UPON THE MEDICAL PROFESSION OF A COMMUNITY.
ALBANY MED ANN 1901;22:1-11.

628. We can only instill principles.

To cover the vast field of medicine in four years is an impossible task. We can only instil principles, put the student in the right path, give him methods, teach him how to study, and early to discern between essentials and non-essentials.

AFTER TWENTY-FIVE YEARS, IN AEQUANIMITAS, 201-2.

629. Prizes are of no value unless they stimulate a better effort.

Prizes and certificates, while of good omen and meaning, more perhaps in the "morn and liquid dew of youth" [from Shakespeare's (1564-1616) *Hamlet*] than at any other period, are of no value unless they impart a stimulus to higher and better effort.

THE RESERVES OF LIFE. ST. MARY'S HOSP GAZ 1907;13:95-8.

630. Study of books alone may spell disaster.

Curiously enough, the student-practitioner may find studiousness to be a stumbling-block in his career. A bookish man may never succeed; deep-versed in books, he may not be able to use his knowledge to practical effect, or, more likely, his failure is not because he has studied books much, but because he has not studied men more.

THE STUDENT LIFE, IN AEQUANIMITAS, 417.

631. The study of anatomy is important.

I am firmly convinced that the best book in medicine is the book of Nature, as writ large in the bodies of men. You remember the answer of the immortal Hunter [John Hunter (1728-1793), English comparative anatomist and surgeon], when asked what books the student should

read in anatomy—he opened the door of the dissecting-room and point-
ed to the tables.

THE NATURAL METHOD OF TEACHING THE SUBJECT OF MEDICINE. JAMA
1901;36:1673-9.

632. The three subjects of training are science, art, and the knowledge of men.

You will be glad to know that the training is in only three subjects—science, art, and the knowledge of men—of equal importance one with
another.

THE RESERVES OF LIFE. ST. MARY'S HOSP GAZ 1907;13:95-8.

633. Repeated experiences are educational.

One evening in the far North-west, beneath the shadows of the Rocky
Mountains we camped beside a small lake from which diverging in all
directions were deep furrows, each one as straight as an arrow, as far as
the eye could reach. They were the deep ruts or tracks which countless
generations of buffaloes had worn in the prairie as they followed each
other to and from the water. In our minds, countless, oft-repeated experiences wear similar ruts in which we find it easiest to travel and out of
which many of us never dream of straying.

THE IMPORTANCE OF POST-GRADUATE STUDY. LANCET 1900;2:73-5.

634. The aviary is a metaphor for how the mind acquires knowledge.

Another especially fortunate comparison is that of the mind to an aviary
which is gradually occupied by different kinds of birds, which corre-
spond to the varieties of knowledge. When we were children the aviary

was empty, and as we grow up we go about "catching" the various kinds of knowledge.

PHYSIC AND PHYSICIANS AS DEPICTED IN PLATO, IN AEQUANIMITAS, 52.

635. High standards of education discourage charlatanism.

The higher the standard of education in a profession the less marked will be the charlatanism, whereas no greater incentive to its development can be found than in sending out from our colleges men who have not had mental training sufficient to enable them to judge between the excellent and the inferior, the sound and the unsound, the true and the half true.

TEACHER AND STUDENT, IN AEQUANIMITAS, 37.

636. What is education?

What, after all, is education but a subtle, slowly-affected change, due to the action upon us of the Externals [environmental influences]; of the written record of the great minds of all ages, of the beautiful and harmonious surroundings of nature and of art, and of the lives, good or ill, of our fellows—these alone educate us, these alone mould the developing minds.

THE LEAVEN OF SCIENCE, IN AEQUANIMITAS, 95.

637. There are three requirements for education.

Given the sacred hunger and proper preliminary training, the student-practitioner requires at least three things with which to stimulate and maintain his education, a notebook, a library, and a quinquennial brain-dusting.

THE STUDENT LIFE, IN AEQUANIMITAS, 411.

638. On-going education in medicine is important.

Here [pathological institute]...the practical man comes for inspiration, for new ideas, and here he finds the touchstone by which he can tell the true in the new. That is to say, if he has sense.

THE PATHOLOGICAL INSTITUTE OF A GENERAL HOSPITAL. GLASGOW MED J
1911;76:321-33.

639. Be sceptical in accepting new claims or data.

A sceptical attitude in these days of hasty observation and of still hastier conclusions is peculiarly appropriate.

ON PHAGOCYTES. MED NEWS [PHILADELPHIA] 1889;54:421-5.

640. The physician needs lifelong training and mental independence.

In no single relation of life does the general practitioner show a more illiberal spirit than in the treatment of himself. I do not refer so much to careless habits of living, to lack of routine in work, or to failure to pay due attention to the business side of the profession—sins which so easily beset him—but I would speak of his failure to realize *first,* the need of a lifelong progressive personal training, and *secondly,* the danger lest in the stress of practice he sacrifice that most precious of all possessions, his mental independence.

CHAUVINISM IN MEDICINE, IN AEQUANIMITAS, 281.

641. Life-long learning is essential.

If the license to practise meant the completion of his education how sad it would be for the practitioner, how distressing to his patients! More clearly than any other the physician should illustrate the truth of Plato's saying that education is a life-long process.

THE IMPORTANCE OF POST-GRADUATE STUDY. LANCET 1900;2:73-5.

642. Chauvinism is a sin.

At any rate, whether he goes abroad or not, let him early escape from the besetting sin of the young physician, *Chauvinism,* that intolerant attitude of mind, which brooks no regard for anything outside his own circle and his own school.

INTERNAL MEDICINE AS A VOCATION, IN AEQUANIMITAS, 135.

Reading, Books, Libraries

643. Bibliomania.

You see here before you a mental, moral, almost, I may say, a physical wreck – and all of your making. Until I became mixed up with you I was really a respectable, God-fearing, industrious, earnest, ardent, enthusiastic, energetic student. Now what am I? A mental wreck, devoted to nothing but your literature. Instead of attending to my duties and attending to my work, in comes every day by the post, and by every post, all this seductive literature with which you have, as you know perfectly well, gradually undermined the mental virility of many a better man than I.

BURROWINGS OF A BOOK-WORM. EGERTON YORRICK DAVIS, GOLDEN, R. THE WORKS OF EGERTON YORRICK DAVIS, MD/SIR WILLIAM OSLER'S ALTER EGO, MONTREAL:OSLER LIBRARY, 1999.

644. To study without patients is not to go to sea.

To study the phenomena of disease without books is to sail an uncharted sea, while to study books without patients is not to go to sea at all.

BOOKS AND MEN, IN AEQUANIMITAS, 210.

645. A library is a corrective of senility.

For the general practitioner a well-used library is one of the few correctives of the premature senility which is so apt to overtake him.

BOOKS AND MEN, IN AEQUANIMITAS, 211.

646. A great library is indispensable.

For the teacher and the worker a great library…is indispensable. They must know the world's best work and know it at once. They mint and make current coin the ore so widely scattered in journals, transactions and monographs.

BOOKS AND MEN, IN AEQUANIMITAS, 210.

647. The joys and benefits of books and libraries are incalculable.

It is hard for me to speak of the value of libraries in terms which would not seem exaggerated. Books have been my delight these thirty years, and from them I have received incalculable benefits.

BOOKS AND MEN, IN AEQUANIMITAS, 210.

648. Read and absorb books.

It is much simpler to buy books than to read them, and easier to read them than to absorb their contents.

THE MEDICAL LIBRARY IN POST-GRADUATE WORK. BRIT MED J 1909;2:925-8.

649. Books are a means to an end.

Some of the best of men have used books the least, and there is good
authority for the statement that shallowness of mind may go with book-
learning,...few will be found to doubt the importance of books as a
means to...the end of all study—the capacity to make a good judgment.

THE MEDICAL LIBRARY IN POST-GRADUATE WORK. BRIT MED J 1909;2:925-8.

650. Books are tools, doctors are craftsmen.

Books are tools, doctors are craftsmen, and so truly as one can measure
the development of any particular handicraft by the variety and complexity of its tools, so we have no better means of judging the intelli-
gence of a profession than by its general collection of books.

THE FUNCTIONS OF A STATE FACULTY. MARYLAND MED J 1897;37:73-7.

651. Books are the tools of the mind.

Books are the tools of the mind, and in a community of progressive
scholars the literature of the world in the different departments of
knowledge must be represented.

ON THE LIBRARY OF A MEDICAL SCHOOL. JOHNS HOPKINS HOSP BULL 1907;18:109-11.

652. Study books and people equally.

Divide your attentions equally between books and men. The strength of
the student of books is to sit still—two or three hours at a stretch—eating the heart out of a subject with pencil and notebook in hand, determined to master the details and intricacies, focussing all your energies on
its difficulties. Get accustomed to test all sorts of book problems and
statements for yourself, and take as little as possible on trust.

THE STUDENT LIFE, IN AEQUANIMITAS, 405.

653. *Without reading, a physician sinks to a low level trade.*

A physician who does not use books and journals, who does not need a library, who does not read one or two of the best weeklies and monthlies, soon sinks to the level of the cross-counter prescriber, and not alone in practice, but in those mercenary feelings and habits which characterize a trade.

THE FUNCTIONS OF A STATE FACULTY. MARYLAND MED J 1897;37:73-7.

654. *Good books influence the business man.*

Teachers and preachers have to know books, but those upon whom their benign influence is most manifest is the ordinary business man to whom they are the very salt of life. A lover of good books is almost always a good man and usually a good citizen—but not always.

BURROWINGS OF A BOOK-WORM. THE WORKS OF EGERTON YORRICK DAVIS, M.D.: SIR WILLIAM OLSER'S ALTER EGO. GOLDEN RL (ED). OSLER LIBRARY, MCGILL UNIVERSITY. MONTREAL, 1999:93-115.

655. *Reading benefits the mind.*

There is no such relaxation for a weary mind as that which is to be had from a good story, a good play or a good essay. It is to the mind what sea breezes and the sunshine of the country are to the body—a change of scene, a refreshment and a solace.

BURROWINGS OF A BOOK-WORM. THE WORKS OF EGERTON YORRICK DAVIS, M.D.: SIR WILLIAM OLSER'S ALTER EGO. GOLDEN RL (ED). OSLER LIBRARY, MCGILL UNIVERSITY. MONTREAL, 1999:93-115.

656. Commune with authors.

It is all a matter of sentiment—so it is, but my very marrow of my bones are full of sentiment, and as I feel toward my blood relations—or some of them!—and to my intimate friends in the flesh, so I feel to these friends in the spirit with whom I am in communion through the medium of the printed page.

BURROWINGS OF A BOOK-WORM. THE WORKS OF EGERTON YORRICK DAVIS, M.D.: SIR WILLIAM OLSER'S ALTER EGO. GOLDEN RL (ED). OSLER LIBRARY, MCGILL UNIVERSITY. MONTREAL, 1999:93-115.

657. Cherish your special books.

I like to think of my few books in an alcove of a fire-proof library of some institution that I love; at the end of an alcove an open fireplace and a few easy chairs, and on the mantelpiece an urn with my ashes and my bust or portrait through which my astral self, like the Bishop of St. Praxed's [from "The Bishop Orders His Tomb at Saint Praxed's Church" by Robert Browning (1812-1889)], could peek at the books I have loved and enjoy the delight with which kindred souls still in the flesh would handle them.

FRANCIS WW. AT OSLER'S SHRINE. BULL MED LIBRARY ASSOC 1937;26:1-8.

658. The Religio Medici should be read by medical students.

The Religio Medici, one of the great English classics [by Thomas Browne (1605-1682), English physician and author], should be in the hands—in the hearts too—of every medical student. As I am on the confessional to-day, I may tell you that no book has had so enduring an influence on my life.

AFTER TWENTY-FIVE YEARS, IN AEQUANIMITAS, 205.

659. Poetry helps to maintain ideals.

A love of books may be the one thing to maintain in him the sentiment of the ideal and it is particularly poetry that has such a value in helping a man to cherish thoughts that lift him above the petty details of life, that strew his path with flowers, that make him hopeful and helpful among his fellows.

BURROWINGS OF A BOOK-WORM. THE WORKS OF EGERTON YORRICK DAVIS, M.D.: SIR WILLIAM OLSER'S ALTER EGO. GOLDEN RL (ED). OSLER LIBRARY, McGILL UNIVERSITY. MONTREAL, 1999:93-115.

660. We need bibliomaniacs.

There is a...class of men in the profession to whom books are dearer than to teachers or practitioners—a small, a silent band.... The profane call them bibliomaniacs, and in truth they are at times irresponsible and do not always know the difference between *meum* [mine] and *tuum* [yours].... Loving books partly for their contents, partly for the sake of the authors, they not alone keep alive the sentiment of historical continuity in the profession.... We need more men of their class, particularly in this country, where every one carries in his pocket the tape-measure of utility.

BOOKS AND MEN, IN AEQUANIMITAS, 212.

661. Bibliomaniacs become obsessive.

In the final stage of the malady...the bibliomaniac haunts the auction rooms and notes with envious eyes the precious volumes as they are handed about for inspection, or chortles with joy as he hears the bids rise higher and higher for some precious treasure already in his possession.

BURROWINGS OF A BOOK-WORM. THE WORKS OF EGERTON YORRICK DAVIS, M.D.: SIR WILLIAM OLSER'S ALTER EGO. GOLDEN RL (ED). OSLER LIBRARY, McGILL UNIVERSITY. MONTREAL, 1999:93-115.

662. Publish your observations.

When you have made and recorded the unusual or original observation, or when you have accomplished a piece of research in laboratory or ward, do not be satisfied with a verbal communication at a medical society. Publish it.

BEAN WB. SIR WILLIAM OSLER: APHORISMS, 60.

663. Your students and disciples will be your greatest honor.

Let every student have full recognition for his work. Never hide the work of others under your own name. Should your assistant make an important observation, let him publish it. Through your students and disciples will come your greatest honour.

THAYER WS. OSLER THE TEACHER, IN OSLER AND OTHER PAPERS, 3, 4.

664. Avoid writing too much or too little.

The difficulty is that the young write too much, the mature write too little. There is too much green fruit sent to market, and the fruit of too many of the fine trees is never plucked at all.

DR. JOHNSTON AS A PHYSICIAN. WASHINGTON MED ANN 1902;1:158-61.

665. Be careful what you write.

The young physician should be careful what and how he writes. Let him take heed to his education, and his reputation will take care of itself.

INTERNAL MEDICINE AS A VOCATION, IN AEQUANIMITAS, 139.

666. Revision is hard.

It is often harder to boil down than to write.

BEAN WB. SIR WILLIAM OSLER: APHORISMS, 60.

667. Osler apologizes for his textbook.

The most unhappy day of my life was when I sold my brains to the publishers.... I must have had neurasthenia or something else, and I beg your pardon for ever having consented to write a book. I have been sorry for students ever since, and trust when Osler goes out of vogue some one will have ready an easier text.

DR. OSLER TO STUDENTS. OKLAHOMA MED J 1900;8:53.

668. The practice of medicine requires reading.

It is astonishing with how little reading a doctor can practise medicine, but it is not astonishing how badly he may do it.

BOOKS AND MEN, IN AEQUANIMITAS, 211.

669. Read in bed every night.

With half an hour's reading in bed every night as a steady practice, the busiest man can get a fair education before the plasma sets in the periganglionic spaces of his grey cortex.

THE MEDICAL LIBRARY IN POST-GRADUATE WORK. BRIT MED J 1909;2:925-8.

670. Have a book open on the dressing table.

A liberal education may be had at a very slight cost of time and money. Well filled though the day be with appointed tasks, to make the best possible use of your one or of your ten talents, rest not satisfied with this professional training, but try to get the education, if not of a scholar, at least of a gentleman. Before going to sleep read for half an hour, and in the morning have a book open on your dressing table. You will be surprised to find how much can be accomplished in the course of a year.

BEDSIDE LIBRARY FOR MEDICAL STUDENTS, IN AEQUANIMITAS, FINAL PAGE.

671. *The habit of reading is mastered early.*

Effort and system gradually train a man's capacity to read intelligently and profitably, but only while the green years are on his head is the habit to be acquired, and in a desultory life, without fixed hours, and with his time at the beck and call of everybody, a man needs a good deal of reserve and determination to maintain it. Once the machinery is started, the effort is not felt in the keen interest in a subject. As Aristotle remarks, "In the case of our habits we are only masters of the beginning, their growth by gradual stages being imperceptible, like the growth of a disease;" and so it is with this habit of reading, of which you are only master at the beginning—once acquired, you are its slave.

THE MEDICAL LIBRARY IN POST-GRADUATE WORK. BRIT MED J 1909;2:925-8.

672. *Live in the ward.*

Live in the ward. Do not waste the hours of daylight in listening to that which you may read by night. But when you have seen, read. And when you can, read the original descriptions of the masters who, with crude methods of study, saw so clearly.

THAYER WS. OSLER THE TEACHER, IN OSLER AND OTHER PAPERS, 1.

673. *Expand your interests.*

Every day do some reading or work apart from your profession. I fully realize, no one more so, how absorbing is the profession of medicine; how applicable to it is what Michelangelo [1475-1564] says: "There are sciences which demand the whole of a man, without leaving the least portion of his spirit free for other distractions;" but you will be a better man and not a worse practitioner for an avocation.

THE STUDENT LIFE, IN AEQUANIMITAS, 414.

674. *Also have an avocation.*

While medicine is to be your vocation, or calling, see to it that you have also an avocation—some intellectual pastime which may serve to keep you in touch with the world of art, of science, or of letters.

AFTER TWENTY-FIVE YEARS, IN AEQUANIMITAS, 204.

675. *Don't relax your studies.*

Men get tired of continuous study, their hearts grow sick under the monotonous daily grind. The more buoyant spirits feel their youth and health strong within them, they relax their rules, they go into society, they begin to spend their evenings in ways more pleasant than in the dry digestion of books; the hard bit of reading is slurred over, the looking up of the lecture notes is put off. "What matter," they think, "it can soon be made up." And so the man becomes an idle man, half-hearted in all that he does, and the grand powers within him lie fallow for want of that earnest persistent exercise of them which alone can bring out their latent strength and make the student all that he might be.

INTRODUCTORY LECTURE, 17.

676. *Overcome the tediousness of study.*

To each of you, gentlemen, I would give the same advice. This feeling of disgust and weariness in study, this disheartening sense of want of progress, is natural; be prepared for it, meet it like a man; the mere effort will draw out the energy you hold in reserve, and you may find, perchance, as many a student has found before you, that the duties taken up with distaste become attractive in the doing of them, if only from that sense of victory over the lower self within us which is, I suppose, one of the most exhilarating and comfortable feelings that any man can possess.

INTRODUCTORY LECTURE, 17-8.

677. *Postgraduate study characterizes medicine.*

Post-graduate study has always been a characteristic feature of our profession.

BEAN WB. SIR WILLIAM OSLER: APHORISMS, 54.

678. *Great ideas from literature inspire.*

But while change is the law, certain great ideas flow fresh through the ages, and control us effectually as in the days of Pericles [5th century B.C. Athenian statesman]. Mankind, it has been said, is always advancing, man is always the same. The love, hope, fear, and faith that make humanity, and the elemental passions of the human heart, remain unchanged, and the secret of inspiration in any literature is the capacity to touch the chord that vibrates in a sympathy that knows nor time nor place.

A WAY OF LIFE, IN A WAY OF LIFE, 249.

679. *Study of the humanities is important to the medical profession.*

But by the neglect of the study of the humanities, which has been far too general, the profession loses a very precious quality.

BRITISH MEDICINE IN GREATER BRITAIN, IN AEQUANIMITAS, 168.

680. *Commune with the saints of humanity.*

The all-important thing is to get a relish for the good company of the race in a daily intercourse with some of the great minds of all ages. Now, in the spring-time of life, pick your intimates among them, and begin a systematic cultivation of their works. Many of you will need a strong leaven to raise you above the dough in which it will be your lot to labour.... Personal contact with men of high purpose and character will help a man to make a start—to have the desire, at least, but in its full-ness this culture—for that word best expresses it—has to be wrought out by each one for himself. Start at once a bed-side library and spend the last half hour of the day in communion with the saints of humanity.

THE MASTER-WORD IN MEDICINE, IN AEQUANIMITAS, 366-7.

681. *The Bible and Shakespeare nourish.*

In life's perspective we seniors are apt to resent that the rising genera-tion should work out its own salvation in ways that are not always our ways, and with thoughts that are not always our thoughts. One thing is in our power, to admix in due proportions with their present somewhat rickety bill of fare the more solid nourishment of the English Bible and of Shakespeare.

WHITE W. OSLER ON SHAKESPEARE, BACON, AND BURTON, WITH A REPRINT OF HIS CREATORS, TRANSMUTERS, AND TRANSMITTERS AS ILLUSTRATED BY SHAKESPEARE, BACON, AND BURTON. BULL HIST MED 1939;7:392-408.

682. *Read the great minds of the immortal dead to gain faith.*

Fifteen or twenty minutes day by day will give you fellowship with the great minds of the race, and little by little as the years pass you extend your friendship with the immortal dead. They will give you faith in your own day.

A WAY OF LIFE, IN A WAY OF LIFE, 248-9.

683. *A periodic "brain dusting" is essential.*

The third essential for the practitioner as a student is the quinquennial brain-dusting, and this will often seem to him the hardest task to carry out.... From the very start begin to save for the trip. Deny yourself all luxuries for it .... Hearken not to the voice of old "Dr. Hayseed," who tells you it will ruin your prospects, and that he "never heard of such a thing" as a young man, not yet five years in practice, taking three months' holiday. To him it seems preposterous. Watch him wince when you say it is a speculation in the only gold mine in which the physician should invest—*Grey Cortex!* What about the wife and babies, if you have them? Leave them! Heavy as are your responsibilities to those nearest and dearest, they are outweighed by the heavier responsibilities to yourself, to the profession, and to the public.

THE STUDENT LIFE, IN AEQUANIMITAS, 414-5.

Examinations

684. Medical students must demonstrate competence to graduate.

The apprentice to get his certificate, the engineer to get his engine, the pilot to get his boat must show practical knowledge and so too must the candidate for the degree in medicine.

UNPUBLISHED DRAFT OF AN ADDRESS TO MEDICAL STUDENTS AT THE UNIVERSITY OF PENNSYLVANIA, 1885. PUBLISHED PRIVATELY BY THE OSLER LIBRARY, MCGILL UNIVERSITY, MONTREAL, 2006.

685. Examinations are a healthy stimulus.

I do not know of any stimulus so healthy as knowledge on the part of the student that he will receive an examination at the end of his course. It gives sharpness to his dissecting knife, heat to his Bunsen burner, a well worn appearance to his stethoscope, and a particular neatliness to his bandaging.

UNPUBLISHED DRAFT OF AN ADDRESS TO MEDICAL STUDENTS AT THE UNIVERSITY OF PENNSYLVANIA, 1885. PUBLISHED PRIVATELY BY THE OSLER LIBRARY, MCGILL UNIVERSITY, MONTREAL, 2006.

686. *Examinations hinder rather than foster learning.*

Perfect happiness for student and teacher will come with the abolition of examinations, which are stumbling blocks and rocks of offence in the pathway of the true student.

AFTER TWENTY-FIVE YEARS, IN AEQUANIMITAS, 202.

687. *Examinations quench the spirit of investigating.*

If we had deliberately set ourselves the task of devising a plan by which this all-precious investigating spirit—which, I repeat, is the very life of the physician—could be quenched, we could not have found anything half so effective as an examination system, which makes the end and object of study the meeting of certain tests; and these, not tests of capacity to do, of capacity to think, but tests of how far a man had himself a Victor-talking-machine [phonograph] or a human monotype on which an examiner might play.

THE RESERVES OF LIFE. ST. MARY'S HOSP GAZ 1907;13:95-8.

688. *The examination should be an accessory in the acquisition of education.*

In its [medicine's] subject matter there is everything in its favour, and it is the easiest possible thing to carry out John Locke's [(1632-1704), English empirical philosopher] primary canon in education—arouse an interest…. It is hard indeed to name a dry subject in the curriculum. And yet in an audience of medical students such a statement nowadays raises a smile. Why? Because we make the examination the end of education, not an accessory in its acquisition. The student is given early the impression that he is in the school to pass certain examinations, and I am afraid the society in which he moves grinds this impression into his soul.

AN INTRODUCTORY ADDRESS ON EXAMINATIONS, EXAMINERS AND EXAMINEES. LANCET 1913;2:1047-50.

689. The student's work should count in his assessment.

Regarding examinations, I have one question to ask—Are they in touch with our system of education? and one suggestion to make—That from the day he enters the school, in laboratory, class-room, and wards, the work of the student should count, and count largely, in the final estimate of his fitness.

AN INTRODUCTORY ADDRESS ON EXAMINATIONS, EXAMINERS AND EXAMINEES. LANCET 1913;2:1047-50.

690. Don't cram for exams.

With too many, unfortunately, working habits are not cultivated until the constraining dread of an approaching examination is felt, when the hopeless attempt is made to cram the work of two years into a six months' session, with results only too evident to your examiners.

INTRODUCTORY LECTURE, 12.

691. Educating for examinations is pernicious.

I have always been opposed to that base and most pernicious system of educating them [students] with a view to examinations, but even the dullest learn how to examine patients, and get familiar with the changing aspects of the important acute diseases.

THE HOSPITAL AS A COLLEGE, IN AEQUANIMITAS, 323.

692. Ensure a sound practice through state boards of medicine.

To move surely [in establishing state licensing boards] we must move slowly, but firmly and fearlessly, confident in the justness of our claims on behalf of the profession and of the public, and animated solely with a desire to secure to the humblest citizen of this great county in the day of his tribulation and in the hour of his need, a skill worthy of the enlightened humanity which we profess, and of the noble calling in which we have the honor to serve.

LICENSE TO PRACTICE. JAMA 1889;12:649-54.

The University

693. *The function of a university is to enlarge knowledge.*

What I mean by the thinking function of a university, is that duty which the professional corps owes to enlarge the boundaries of human knowledge. Work of this sort makes a university great, and alone enables it to exercise a wide influence on the minds of men.

TEACHING AND THINKING: THE TWO FUNCTIONS OF A MEDICAL SCHOOL, IN A WAY OF LIFE, 202.

694. *A university has two purposes.*

A great university has a dual function, to teach and to think.

TEACHING AND THINKING, IN AEQUANIMITAS, 120.

695. *Teaching medicine is one of the noblest functions of the university.*

In teaching men what disease is, how it may be prevented, and how it may be cured, a University is fulfilling one of its very noblest functions.

TEACHING AND THINKING, IN AEQUANIMITAS, 125.

696. Outstanding teachers with practical experience should be in charge of university departments.

The aim of a school should be to have these departments in the charge of men who have, first, *enthusiasm,* that deep love of a subject, that desire to teach and extend it without which all instruction becomes cold and lifeless; secondly, *a full personal knowledge of the branch taught;* not a second-hand information derived from books but the living experience derived from experimental and practical work in the best laboratories. Thirdly, men are required who have a *sense of obligation,* that feeling which impels a teacher to be also a contributor, and to add to the stores from which he so freely draws.

TEACHER AND STUDENT, IN AEQUANIMITAS, 29.

697. The glory of the university lies in its faculty.

The great possession of any University is its great names. It is not the "pride, pomp and circumstance" [from Shakespeare's (1564-1616) *Othello*] of an institution which bring honour, not its wealth, nor the number of its schools, not the students who throng its halls, but the *men* who have trodden in its service the thorny road through toil, even through hate, to the serene abode to Fame, climbing "like stars to their appointed height." [from *Adonais* by Percy Bysshe Shelley (1792-1822)] These bring glory, and it should thrill the heart of every alumnus.

AEQUANIMITAS, IN AEQUANIMITAS, 9.

698. Without teaching, an institution is not first class.

The work of an institution in which there is no teaching is rarely first class. There is not that keen interest nor the thorough study of the cases, nor amid the exigencies of the busy life is the hospital physician able to escape clinical slovenliness unless he teaches and in turn is taught by assistants and students. It is, I think, safe to say that in a hospital with students in the wards the patients are more carefully looked after, their diseases are more fully studied and fewer mistakes made.

On the Need of a Radical Reform in Our Methods of Teaching Senior
Students. Med News [New York] 1903;82:49-53.

699. *The university must select teachers who have knowledge, ideas, and ambition.*

In a school which...wishes to do thinking as well as teaching, men must be selected who are not only thoroughly *au courant* with the best work in their department the world over, but who also have ideas, with ambition and energy to put them into force—men who can add each one in his sphere, to the store of the world's knowledge. Men of this stamp alone confer greatness upon a university.

Teaching and Thinking, in Aequanimitas, 128.

700. *Without the personal influence of teachers, a university is petrified.*

An academical system without the personal influence of teachers upon pupils, is an Arctic winter; it will create an ice-bound, petrified, cast-iron University, and nothing else.

Teacher and Student, in Aequanimitas, 26.

701. *Faculties should have their ferment.*

A faculty without its troubles is always in a bad way—the water should be stirred. Some ferment should be brewing; the young men should always be asking for improvements, to which the old men would object.

Impressions of Paris. I. Teachers and Students. JAMA 1909;52:701-73.

702. Fellowships and scholarships support bright young physicians and stimulate faculty.

With a system of fellowships and research scholarships a university may have a body of able young men, who on the outposts of knowledge are exploring, surveying, defining and correcting.... Surrounded by a group of bright young minds, well trained in advanced methods, not only is the professor himself stimulated to do his best work, but he has to keep far afield and to know what is stirring in every part of his own domain.

TEACHING AND THINKING, IN AEQUANIMITAS, 128-9.

703. What a hospital should be.

The type of school I have always felt the Hospital should be: a place of refuge for the sick poor of the city—a place where the best that is known is taught to a group of the best students—a place where new thought is materialized in research—a school where men are encouraged to base the art upon the science of medicine—a fountain to which teachers in every subject would come for inspiration—a place with a hearty welcome to every practitioner who seeks help—a consulting center for the whole country in cases of obscurity.

BEAN WB. SIR WILLIAM OSLER: APHORISMS, 51.

Teachers and Teaching

704. Instructors are also guardians.

Our duties over as your instructors, we become as examiners, guardians, of a double trust – the honor of the University and the well-being of the citizens and to these we must be as faithful as we have endeavored to be in our capacity as your teachers.

Unpublished draft of an address to medical students at the University of Pennsylvania, 1885. Published privately by The Osler Library, McGill University, Montreal, 2006.

705. *Teachers are responsible for the mistakes of their students.*

The errors of incompetency, the fatal mistakes of culpable ignorance may be morally laid at the doors of men who allow graduates to go forth incapable of meeting the common accident and diseases of life.

Unpublished draft of an address to medical students at the University of Pennsylvania, 1885. Published privately by The Osler Library, McGill University, Montreal, 2006.

706. *The value of lectures is controversial.*

Of the precise value of the didactic lectures in a medical course, there are differences of opinion. In the universal rage for the practical, we hear murmurs of discontent and the opinion is even openly expressed that from lectures not more can be gathered than from good text books.

Unpublished draft of an address to medical students at the University of Pennsylvania, 1885. Published privately by The Osler Library, McGill University, Montreal, 2006.

707. *We believe most what we hear.*

As a rule, there can be no question of the superiority of the instruction given by the living, the vox viva, over that by the reading of textbooks. Somehow we have more faith in what is told us than in what we read.

Unpublished draft of an address to medical students at the University of Pennsylvania, 1885. Published privately by The Osler Library, McGill University, Montreal, 2006.

708. Clinical experience adds value to a lecture.

The personal experience of the lecturer impresses the learner and gives a special value to these courses which are greatly determined by men with a wide and varied acquaintance with disease.

UNPUBLISHED DRAFT OF AN ADDRESS TO MEDICAL STUDENTS AT THE UNIVERSITY OF PENNSYLVANIA, 1885. PUBLISHED PRIVATELY BY THE OSLER LIBRARY, MCGILL UNIVERSITY, MONTREAL, 2006.

709. The natural method of teaching begins and ends with the patient.

In what may be called the natural method of teaching the student begins with the patient, continues with the patient, and ends his studies with the patient, using books and lectures as tools, as means to an end.

THE HOSPITAL AS A COLLEGE, IN AEQUANIMITAS, 315.

710. Teaching medicine requires patients.

The dissociation of student and patient is a legacy of the pernicious system of theoretical teaching.

ON THE NEED OF A RADICAL REFORM IN OUR METHODS OF TEACHING SENIOR STUDENTS. MED NEWS [NEW YORK] 1903;82:49-53.

711. The effective teacher is remembered.

In the hurly-burly of to-day, when the competition is so keen...it is well for young men to remember that no bubble is so iridescent or floats longer than that blown by the successful teacher.

THE PATHOLOGICAL INSTITUTE OF A GENERAL HOSPITAL. GLASGOW MED J 1911;76:321-33.

712. *The successful teacher and the student are close.*

The successful teacher is no longer on a height, pumping knowledge at high pressure into passive receptacles…. When a simple, earnest spirit animates a college, there is no appreciable interval between the teacher and the taught—both are in the same class, the one a little more advanced than the other. So animated, the student feels that he has joined a family whose honour is his honour, whose welfare is his own, and whose interests should be his first consideration.

THE STUDENT LIFE, IN AEQUANIMITAS, 399-400.

713. *Teachers are also students.*

It goes without saying that no man can teach successfully who is not at the same time a student.

THE STUDENT LIFE, IN AEQUANIMITAS, 419.

714. *Students should take pride in their teachers.*

What, for example, is more proper than the pride which we feel in our teachers, in the university from which we have graduated, in the hospital at which we have been trained? He is a "poor sort" who is free from such feelings, which only manifest a proper loyalty.

CHAUVINISM IN MEDICINE, IN AEQUANIMITAS, 279.

715. *Teachers should provide students with methods and patients.*

A teacher of medicine should ever have two objects in view: first, to give to the student, in the Art and in the Science, good methods; and secondly, to enable him to follow closely and accurately as many cases of disease as possible.

ON THE STUDY OF PNEUMONIA. ST. PAUL MED J 1899;1:5-9.

716. An enthusiastic teacher is contagious.

The dry formal lecture never, or at any rate rarely, touches the heart, but it is in [the] conversational method of the seminar, or in the quiet evening at home, with a select group and a few good editions of a favorite author, that the enthusiasm of the teacher becomes contagious.

BURROWINGS OF A BOOK-WORM. THE WORKS OF EGERTON YORRICK DAVIS, M.D.: SIR WILLIAM OSLER'S ALTER EGO. GOLDEN RL (ED). OSLER LIBRARY, MCGILL UNIVERSITY. MONTREAL, 1999:93-115.

717. The responsibilities of a good teacher are several.

Punctuality, the class first, always and at all times; the best that a man has in him, nothing less; the best the profession has on the subject, nothing less; fresh energies and enthusiasm in dealing with dry details; animated, unselfish devotion to all alike; tender consideration for his assistants— these are some of the fruits of a keen sense of responsibility in a good teacher.

THE STUDENT LIFE, IN AEQUANIMITAS, 420.

718. Lectures can pain the buttocks.

Superfluity of lecturing causes ischial bursitis.

BEAN WB. SIR WILLIAM OSLER: APHORISMS, 46.

719. Teaching on the wards is a great pleasure.

The best life of the teacher is in supervising the personal daily contact of patient with student in the wards.

THE SCHOOL OF PHYSIC, DUBLIN, IN MEN AND BOOKS, 29.

720. Teaching digestible facts is taxing.

To winnow the wheat from the chaff and to prepare it in an easily digested shape for the tender stomachs of the first and second year students taxes the resources of the most capable teacher.

AFTER TWENTY-FIVE YEARS, IN AEQUANIMITAS, 199.

721. It is futile to teach all to all students.

Then let us boldly acknowledge the futility of attempting to teach all to all students.... It is barbaric cruelty with so much ahead to burden the mind with minutiae which have only a Chinese value—a titanic test of memory. To schedule a minimum of the essentials should not be difficult, once the great principle is acknowledged that in all departments of the curriculum only a few subjects can be mastered thoroughly.

AN INTRODUCTORY ADDRESS ON EXAMINATIONS, EXAMINERS AND EXAMINEES. LANCET 1913;2:1047-50.

722. The teacher's life has three periods.

The teacher's life should have three periods, study until twenty-five, investigation until forty, profession until sixty, at which age I would have him retired on a double allowance.

THE FIXED PERIOD, IN AEQUANIMITAS, 383.

723. Students prevent staleness in teachers.

But for the majority, daily contact with students, and a little of the routine of teaching, keep us in touch with the common clay and are the best preservatives against that staleness so apt to come as a blight upon the pure researcher.

BEAN WB. SIR WILLIAM OSLER: APHORISMS, 47.

724. The best teacher may not be an investigator and vice versa.

Teachers who teach current knowledge are not necessarily investigators; many have not had the needful training; others have not the needful time. The very best instructor for students may have no conception of the higher lines of work in his branch, and contrariwise, how many brilliant investigators have been wretched teachers?

TEACHING AND THINKING, IN AEQUANIMITAS, 128.

725. Good teachers teach the best information and create new knowledge

The function of the teacher is to teach and to propagate the best that is known and taught in the world. To teach the current knowledge of the subject he professes—sifting, analyzing, assorting, laying down principles. To propagate, i.e., to multiply, facts on which to base principles—experimenting, searching, testing. The best that is known and taught in the world—nothing less can satisfy a teacher worthy of the name.

TEACHER AND STUDENT, IN AEQUANIMITAS, 27.

726. Medical schools are made up of diverse teaching talents.

Professors similarly may be divided into four classes. There is, first, the man who can think but who has neither tongue nor technique. Though useless for the ordinary student, he may be the leaven of a faculty and the chief glory of his university. A second variety is the phonographic professor, who can talk but who can neither think nor work. Under the old régime he repeated year by year the same lecture. A third is the man who has technique but who can neither talk nor think; and a fourth is the rare professor who can do all three—think, talk and work. With these types fairly represented in a faculty, the diversities of gifts only serving to illustrate the wide spirit of the teacher, the Dean at least should feel happy.

AFTER TWENTY-FIVE YEARS, IN AEQUANIMITAS, 199-200.

727. We need to teach teachers.

One great difficulty is that only a few are really competent to teach students the art. We need a school of medical pedagogy in which able young men, aspiring to the position of teachers, could be taught proper methods. We still have the primitive belief that any man is good enough to be a teacher, either of boys or of men.

THE RESERVES OF LIFE. ST. MARY'S HOSP GAZ 1907;13:95-8.

728. Teachers should also practice medicine.

I cannot imagine anything more subversive to the highest ideal of a clinical school than to hand over young men who are to be our best practitioners to a group of teachers who are *ex officio* out of touch with the conditions under which these young men will live. The clinical teachers belong to the fighting line of the profession, whose ambitions and activities they should share and direct.

ON FULL-TIME CLINICAL TEACHING IN MEDICAL SCHOOLS. CAN MED ASSOC J
1962;87:762-5.

729. Recruit fit professors.

The professoriate of the profession, the most mobile column of its great army, should be recruited with the most zealous regard to fitness, irrespective of local conditions that are apt to influence the selection.

CHAUVINISM IN MEDICINE, IN AEQUANIMITAS, 280.

730. All physicians have an obligation to teach.

The same obligation rests on him to know and to teach the best that is known and taught in the world—on the surgeon the obligation to know thoroughly the scientific principles on which his art is based, to be a master in the technique of his handicraft, ever studying, modifying, improving;—on the physician, the obligation to study the natural history of diseases and the means for their prevention, to know the true value of regimen, diet and drugs in their treatment, ever testing, devising, thinking;—and upon both, to teach to their students habits of reliance, and to be to them examples of gentleness, forbearance and courtesy in dealing with their suffering brethren.

TEACHER AND STUDENT, IN AEQUANIMITAS, 30-1.

731. Provide support for faculty to prevent burnout.

One of the chief difficulties in the way of advanced work is the stress of routine class and laboratory duties, which often sap the energies of men capable of higher things. To meet this difficulty it is essential, first, to give the professors plenty of assistance, so that they will not be worn out with teaching; and, secondly, to give encouragement to graduates and others to carry on researches under their direction.

TEACHING AND THINKING, IN AEQUANIMITAS, 128.

732. Faculty are woefully underpaid.

Owing these men [faculty] an enormous debt, since we reap where they have sown, and garner the fruits of their husbandry, what do we give them in return? Too often beggarly salaries and an exacting routine of teaching which saps all initiative. Both in the United States and Canada the professoriate as a class, the men who live by college teaching, is wretchedly underpaid.

AFTER TWENTY-FIVE YEARS, IN AEQUANIMITAS, 197.

733. Don't stay in the same pasture too long.

The question may be asked—whether as professors we do not stay too long in one place. It passes my persimmon to tell how some good men—even lovable and righteous men in other respects—have the hardihood to stay in the same position for twenty-five years! To a man of active mind too long attachment to one college is apt to breed self-satisfaction, to narrow his outlook, to foster a local spirit, and to promote senility.... We are apt to grow stale and thin mentally if kept too long in the same pasture.

THE FIXED PERIOD, IN AEQUANIMITAS, 377.

734. Faculty are bewildered by the complexity and rapidity of change.

The actual care of the sick, once our sole duty, is now supplemented by such a host of other activities, social, scientific, and administrative, that an ever-increasing number of our members have nothing to do with patients as such.... Everywhere increased complexity and mind-burdening terminology. What is the teacher to do? And more important, what can the poor student do, confronted with so much new knowledge and Rabelaisian [François Rabelais (1494?-1553), French humorist and satirist] onomatomania?

AN INTRODUCTORY ADDRESS ON EXAMINATIONS, EXAMINERS AND EXAMINEES. LANCET 1913;2:1047-50.

735. Be ready to say "I do not know."

I have learned since to be a better student, and to be ready to say to my fellow students "I do not know."

AFTER TWENTY-FIVE YEARS, IN AEQUANIMITAS, 195.

736. Osler valued his teaching above all.

I desire no other epitaph...than the statement that I taught medical students in the wards, as I regard this as by far the most useful and important work I have been called upon to do.

THE FIXED PERIOD, IN AEQUANIMITAS, 390.

7

Men and Women, Aging, History

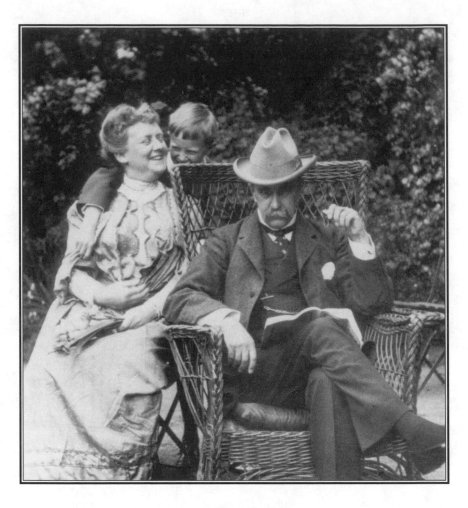

William and Grace Osler with son Revere, age 10,
at 13 Norham Gardens, Oxford, in 1905.
(Courtesy of the Osler Library of the History of Medicine,
Montreal, Quebec, Canada.)

Men and Women, Aging, History

Men and Women

737. *There are two primal passions of man.*

The natural man has only two primal passions, to get and to beget—to get the means of sustenance and...to beget his kind.

SCIENCE AND IMMORTALITY, 10.

738. *Passion is a heavy burden*

The other primal instinct is the heavy burden of the flesh which Nature puts on all of us to ensure a continuation of the species. To drive Plato's team taxes the energies of the best of us. One of the horses is a raging, untamed devil, who can only be brought into subjection by hard fighting and severe training. This much you all know as men: once the bit is between his teeth the black steed Passion will take the white horse Reason with you and the chariot rattling over the rocks to perdition [from Plato's *Phaedrus*].

A WAY OF LIFE, IN A WAY OF LIFE, 245.

739. *Man is significant—to himself.*

Knowing not whence he came, why he is here, or whither he is going, man feels himself of supreme importance, and certainly is of interest—to himself. Let us hope that he has indeed a potency and importance out of all proportion to his somatic insignificance.

THE EVOLUTION OF MODERN MEDICINE, 2.

740. *Cheerfulness annoys the grouchy.*

A cheerful man at the breakfast table is a great annoyance to his grouchy neighbor.

BEAN WB. SIR WILLIAM OSLER: APHORISMS, 85.

741. *Friendship is essential for happiness.*

In the life of a young man the most essential thing for happiness is the gift of friendship.

VALLERY-RADOT R. THE LIFE OF PASTEUR (INTRODUCTION BY WILLIAM OSLER). LONDON: CONSTABLE AND CO., 1911, 9-22.

742. *The majority do not receive appreciation for their work.*

Upon men obviously striving to be taken at their own valuation the world has no mercy; now and again one wins out, but the majority form a battered band whose work and worth never receive a due mead of appreciation. It is the careless sinner who goes awhistling and working through life, caring not for what the world thinks, who gets more than his due.

PROFESSOR WESLEY MILLS. CAN MED ASSOC J 1915;5:338-41.

743. The human mind is full of delusions.

The history of the progress of the human mind is a history of a struggle with its delusions.

THE POWDER OF SYMPATHY. SIR KENELM DIGBY'S POWDER OF SYMPATHY: AN UNFINISHED ESSAY BY SIR WILLIAM OSLER. LOS ANGELES: PLANTIN PRESS, 1972:1.

744. World War I reveals the dark side of humanity.

In the midst of this great struggle [World War I] we stand aghast at the carnage—at the sacrifice of so many lives in their prime—"That many men so beautiful,/And they all dead did lie." [from *The Rime of the Ancient Mariner* by Samuel Taylor Coleridge (1772-1834)] The bitterness of it comes home every morning as we read in the Role of Honour the names of the much loved sons of dear friends. Strange that man who dominates Nature has so departed from Nature as to be the only animal to wage relentless war on his own species.

THE WAR AND TYPHOID FEVER. BRIT MED J 1914;2:909-13.

745. The history of the race is a grim record of barbarism.

The history of the race is a grim record of passions and ambitions, of weaknesses and vanities, a record, too often, of barbaric inhumanity; and even to-day, when philosophers would have us believe his thoughts had widened, he is ready as of old to shut the gates of mercy, and to let loose the dogs of war.

DOCTOR AND NURSE, IN AEQUANIMITAS, 17.

746. *Civilization is a fringe on history.*

Civilization is but a filmy fringe on the history of man.

THE EVOLUTION OF MODERN MEDICINE, 2.

747. *The inhumanity of man to man is the greatest atrocity.*

The history of man is a story of a great martyrdom—plague, pestilence and famine, battle and murder, crimes unspeakable, tortures inconceivable, and the inhumanity of man to man has even outdone what appear to be atrocities in nature.

MAN'S REDEMPTION OF MAN. NEW YORK: PAUL B. HOEBER, 1915:9-10.

748. *Intolerance is to be cursed.*

Breathes there a man with soul so dead that it does not glow at the thought of what the men of his blood have done and suffered to make his country what it is?…What I inveigh against is a cursed spirit of intolerance, conceived in distrust and bred in ignorance, that makes the mental attitude perennially antagonistic, even bitterly antagonistic to everything foreign, that subordinates everywhere the race to the nation, forgetting the higher claims of human brotherhood.

CHAUVINISM IN MEDICINE, IN AEQUANIMITAS, 271.

749. *Advice is sought to confirm.*

Advice is sought to confirm a position already taken.

BEAN WB. SIR WILLIAM OSLER: APHORISMS, 91.

750. *Women can fool men but not always women.*

Women can fool men always, women only sometimes.

NURSE AND PATIENT, IN AEQUANIMITAS, 152.

751. *Marry the right woman.*

This well-drawn character [Tertius Lydgate, an ambitious young physician in George Eliot's *Middlemarch* (1871-72)] may be studied with advantage by the physician; one of the most important lessons to be gathered from it is—marry the right woman!

INTERNAL MEDICINE AS A VOCATION, IN AEQUANIMITAS, 136.

752. *Unmarried women must channel their energies or they may be dangerous.*

I do not know at what age one dare call a woman a spinster. I will put it, perhaps rashly, at twenty-five. Now, at that critical period a woman who has not to work for her living, who is without urgent domestic ties, is very apt to become a dangerous element unless her energies and emotions are diverted in a proper channel.

NURSE AND PATIENT, IN AEQUANIMITAS, 157.

753. *Avoid wine and women.*

Avoid wine and women—choose a freckle-faced girl for a wife; they are invariably more amiable.

BEAN WB. SIR WILLIAM OSLER: APHORISMS, 70.

754. *Most women are tactful.*

It is one of the greatest blessings that so many women are so full of tact. The calamity happens when a woman who has all the other riches of life just lacks that one thing.

BEAN WB. SIR WILLIAM OSLER: APHORISMS, 119.

755. Women should receive the best medical education.

How far it may be expedient to encourage women to enter the medical profession, the work of which is often disagreeable and always laborious, is a question which receives very diverse answers; but the right of women to study medicine is now granted on all sides.... If any woman feels that the medical profession is her vocation, no obstacle should be placed in the way of her obtaining the best possible education, and every facility should be offered, so that, as a practitioner, she should have a fair start in the race.

ON THE OPENING OF THE JOHNS HOPKINS MEDICAL SCHOOL TO WOMEN. CENTURY MAG 1891;41:635.

756. There is no longer hostility to women in medicine.

When Mary Putnam [(1842-1906), New York physician, author, and social reformer] returned from Europe with a Paris medical degree, and a training in scientific medicine unusual at that date [1871] even among men, the status of women as doctors was still unsettled. Between the open hostility of the many and the half-hearted sympathy of the few, the position of those in the profession was a most unenviable one. That in the past quarter of a century the long battle has been won is due less to a growing tolerance among physicians at large, less to the persistence with which obvious rights have been asserted, than to the presence of a few notable figures who have demonstrated the capacity of women for the highest intellectual development and who have compelled recognition by the character of work accomplished in the science and in the art of medicine.

IN MEMORIAM OF MARY PUTNAM JACOBI. NY MED REC 1907;66:3-8.

757. Women are better adapted to scientific work.

That a larger proportion of women than of men are unfit for practice, will, I think, be acknowledged; on the other hand, a relatively larger proportion of the former are adapted to scientific work, and it is a most encouraging feature to see so many women taking up laboratory life. In chemistry, histology, pathology, embryology, bacteriology, and even in anatomy, the work which they are doing is everywhere attracting attention. Here they meet men as equals, since what they lack in initiative and independence is counterbalanced by a more delicate technique, a greater patience with minutiae, and a greater mastery of detail. In the scientific life, too, woman escapes those little rebuffs and slights so trying to a sensitive nature, and to which it is not good for a woman to become so hardened that they do not hurt.

IN MEMORIAM OF MARY PUTNAM JACOBI. NY MED REC 1907;66:3-8.

758. A woman physician of greatness will arrive.

For years I have been waiting the advent of the modern Trotula [a woman or women associated with the medical school at Salerno in Italy during the Middle Ages], a woman in the profession with an intellect so commanding that she will rank with the Harveys, the Hunters, and Pasteurs; the Virchows, and the Listers. That she has not yet arisen is no reflection on the small band of women physicians who have joined our ranks in the last fifty years. Stars of the first magnitude are rare, but that such a one will arise among woman physicians I have not the slightest doubt. And let us be thankful that when she comes she will not have to waste her precious energies in the worry of a struggle for recognition.

CUSHING H. THE LIFE OF SIR WILLIAM OSLER, VOL. 2, 76.

Aging and "The Fixed Period"*

759. The first fixed idea: Men above 40 are relatively useless.

I have two fixed ideas well known to my friends, harmless obsessions with which I sometimes bore them, but which have a direct bearing on this important problem. The first is the comparative uselessness of men above forty years of age. This may seem shocking, and yet read aright the world's history bears out the statement. Take the sum of human achievement in action, in science, in art, in literature—subtract the work of the men above forty, and while we should miss great treasures, even priceless treasures, we would practically be where we are to-day. It is difficult to name a great and far-reaching conquest of the mind which has not been given to the world by a man on whose back the sun was still shining.

THE FIXED PERIOD, IN AEQUANIMITAS, 381.

760. The second fixed idea: Men above sixty should retire.

My second fixed idea is the uselessness of men above sixty years of age, and the incalculable benefit it would be in commercial, political and in professional life if, as a matter of course, men stopped work at this age.... That incalculable benefits might follow such a scheme is apparent to any one who, like myself, is nearing the limit, and who has made a careful study of the calamities which may befall men during the seventh and eighth decades.

THE FIXED PERIOD, IN AEQUANIMITAS, 382.

---

*Editors' note: Osler maintained that most significant contributions to human knowledge and culture are made before the age of 40 years. In a farewell address in 1905, Osler, then 56 and retiring from his stressful academic life at Johns Hopkins to become the Regius professor at Oxford, alluded to one of Anthony Trollope's (1815-1882) novels, *The Fixed Period*. The satirical plot of Trollope's novel hinges on a scheme whereby men retire at the age of 67 for a year of contemplation before death by euthanasia. The press sensationalized Osler's allusion and misrepresented him as being unfriendly to the elderly. For a while, "to Oslerize" was used as a synonym for euthanasia.

761. The great advances are accomplished between ages twenty-five and forty.

The effective, moving, vitalizing work of the world is done between the ages of twenty-five and forty—these fifteen golden years of plenty, the anabolic or constructive period, in which there is always a balance in the mental bank and the credit is still good.

THE FIXED PERIOD, IN AEQUANIMITAS, 381.

762. Evil mistakes and drivel are mostly produced by sexagenarians.

As it can be maintained that all the great advances have come from men under forty, so the history of the world shows that a very large proportion of the evils may be traced to the sexagenarians—nearly all the great mistakes politically and socially, all of the worst poems, most of the bad pictures, a majority of the bad novels, not a few of the bad sermons and speeches.

THE FIXED PERIOD, IN AEQUANIMITAS, 382-3.

763. No one is indispensable.

It is strange of how slight value is the unit in a great system. A man may have built up a department and have gained a certain following, local or general; nay, more, he may have had a special value for his mental and moral qualities, and his fission may leave a scar, even an aching scar, but it is not for long. Those of us accustomed to the process know that the organism as a whole feels it about as much as a big polyzoon when a colony breaks off, or a hive of bees after a swarm—'tis not indeed always a calamity, oftentimes it is a relief.

THE FIXED PERIOD, IN AEQUANIMITAS, 376.

764. *Increasing demands come with success.*

After years of hard work, at the very time when a man's energies begin to flag, and when he feels the need of more leisure, the conditions and surroundings that have made him what he is and that have moulded his character and abilities into something useful in the community—these very circumstances ensure an ever increasing demand upon them.

THE FIXED PERIOD, IN AEQUANIMITAS, 375.

765. *Benefits should accompany old age.*

The things that should accompany old age: fairly good health to the end, an unceasing interest in life, and the affectionate esteem of a large circle of friends.

SAMUEL WILKS, IN MEN AND BOOKS, 6.

766. *The old may resent the young.*

In life's perspective we seniors are apt to resent that the rising generation should work out its own salvation in ways that are not always our ways, and with thoughts that are not always our thoughts.

CREATORS, TRANSMUTERS, AND TRANSMITTERS, IN A WAY OF LIFE, 7.

767. *Learn to recognize old fogeyism.*

Would you recognize the signs by which in man or institution you may recognize old fogeyism? They are three things: first, a state of blissful happiness and contentment with things as they are; secondly, a supreme conviction that the condition of other people and other institutions is one of pitiable inferiority; and thirdly, a fear of change, which not alone perplexes but appals.

THE IMPORTANCE OF POST-GRADUATE STUDY. LANCET 1900;2:73-7.

768. Conservation and fogeyism are different.

Conservatism and old fogeyism are totally different things; the motto of the one is "Prove all things and hold fast that which is good" and of the other "Prove nothing but hold fast that which is old." [from *The First Epistle of Paul the Apostle to Timothy*, I Timothy 1:8]

THE IMPORTANCE OF POST-GRADUATE STUDY. LANCET 1900;2:73-7.

769. The aging physician professor is less able to adapt to change.

From one who, like themselves, has passed *la crise de quarante ans*, the seniors present will pardon a few plain remarks upon the disadvantages to a school of having too many men of mature, not to say riper, years. Insensibly, in the fifth and sixth decades, there begins to creep over most of us a change, noted physically among other ways the silvering of the hair and that lessening of elasticity, which impels a man to open rather than to vault a five-barred gate. It comes to all sooner or later; to some it is only too painfully evident, to others it comes unconsciously, with no pace perceived. And with most of us this physical change has its mental equivalent, not necessarily accompanied by loss of the powers of application or of judgment; on the contrary, often the mind grows clearer and the memory more retentive, but the change is seen in a weakened receptivity and in an inability to adapt oneself to an altered intellectual environment. It is this loss of mental elasticity which makes men over forty so slow to receive new truths.

TEACHER AND STUDENT, IN AEQUANIMITAS, 31-2.

770. Post-graduate study is an antidote to early senility.

Men above forty are rarely pioneers, rarely the creators in science or in literature. The work of the world has been done by men who had not reached *la crise de guarante ans* [the crisis of forty years; mid-life crisis].

And in our profession wipe out, with but few exceptions, the contributions of men above this age and we remain essentially as we are. Once across this line we teachers and consultants are in constant need of post-graduate study as an antidote against premature senility. Daily contact with the bright young minds of our associates and assistants, the mental friction of medical societies, and travel are important aids.

THE IMPORTANCE OF POST-GRADUATE STUDY. LANCET 1900;2:73-5.

History

771. The past is always with us.

The past is always with us, never to be escaped; it alone is enduring; but, amidst the changes and chances which succeed one another so rapidly in this life, we are apt to live too much for the present and too much in the future.

AEQUANIMITAS, IN AEQUANIMITAS, 8-9.

772. Inspiration comes from remembering the past.

In the continual remembrance of a glorious past individuals and nations find their noblest inspiration, and if to-day this inspiration, so valuable for its own sake, so important in its associations, is weakened, is it not because in the strong dominance of the individual, so characteristic of a democracy, we have lost the sense of continuity?

THE LEAVEN OF SCIENCE, IN AEQUANIMITAS, 75.

773. Contemplate and learn from the past.

In the records of no other profession is there to be found so large a number of men who have combined intellectual pre-eminence with nobility of character. This higher education so much needed to-day is not given in the school, is not to be bought in the marketplace, but it has to be wrought out in each one of us for himself; it is the silent influence of character on character and in no way more potent than in the contemplation of the lives of the great and good of the past, in no way more than in "the touch divine of noble natures gone."

BOOKS AND MEN, IN A WAY OF LIFE, 38.

774. Medical history is valuable in problem solving.

By the historical method alone can many problems in medicine be approached profitably.

BOOKS AND MEN, IN AEQUANIMITAS, 212-3.

775. Students need contact with the humanities.

The Humanities bring the student into contact with the master minds who gave us these things [the philosophies, the models of our literature, the ideals of democratic freedom, the fine and technical arts, the fundamentals of science, the basis of our law]...with the dead who never die, with those immortal lives "not of now, or of yesterday but which always were."

THE OLD HUMANITIES AND THE NEW SCIENCE. BRIT MED J 1919;2:1-7.

776. Venerate great men.

Of the altruistic instincts veneration is not the most highly developed at the present day, but I hold strongly with the statement that it is the sign of a dry age when the great men of the past are held in light esteem.

THE FUNCTIONS OF A STATE FACULTY. MARYLAND MED J 1897;37:73-7.

777. Be a hero worshiper

It helps a man immensely to be a bit of a hero-worshipper, and the stories of the lives of the masters of medicine do much to stimulate our ambition and rouse our sympathies.

CHAUVINISM IN MEDICINE, IN AEQUANIMITAS, 273.

778. Understand great figures in the context of the past.

To understand the old writers one must see as they saw, feel as they felt, believe as they believed—and this is hard, indeed impossible! We may get near them by asking the Spirit of the Age in which they lived to enter in and dwell with us, but it does not always come.... Each generation has its own problems to face, looks at truth from a special focus and does not see quite the same outlines as any other.

THE EVOLUTION OF MODERN MEDICINE, 218.

779. See the future within the context of the past.

The secret of success in an institution...is to blend the old with the new, the past with the present in due proportion, and it is not difficult if we follow Emerson's [1803-1882] counsel: "We cannot overstate," he says, "our debt to the past, but the moment has the supreme claim; the sole terms on which the past can become ours are its subordination to the present."

CUSHING H. THE LIFE OF SIR WILLIAM OSLER, VOL. 2, 177.

780. History is the study of individuals.

History is simply the biography of the mind of man; and our interest in history, and its educational value to us, is directly proportionate to the completeness of our study of the individuals through whom this mind has been manifested.

HARVEY AND HIS DISCOVERY, IN AN ALABAMA STUDENT, 296.

781. *Our memories of a man may depend on trifles.*

It is strange how the memory of a man may float to posterity on what he would have himself regarded as the most trifling of his works.

JEAN ASTRUC AND THE HIGHER CRITICISM, IN MEN AND BOOKS, 7.

782. *Literature requires a historical context.*

To separate in literature the quick from the dead is one of the functions of a well-ordered library; but much that we carelessly regard as dead is magnetized into life when put in its historical relation.

THE FIRST PRINTED DOCUMENTS RELATING TO MODERN SURGICAL ANAESTHESIA.

ANN MED HIST 1917:329-32.

783. *The Hippocratic foundations of modern medicine are essential.*

The critical sense and sceptical attitude of the Hippocratic school laid the foundations of modern medicine on broad lines, and we owe to it: *first,* the emancipation of medicine from the shackles of priestcraft and of caste; *secondly,* the conception of medicine as an art based on accurate observation, and as a science, an integral part of the science of man and of nature; *thirdly,* the high moral ideals, expressed in...the Hippocratic oath; and *fourthly,* the conception and realization of medicine as the profession of a cultivated gentleman. No other profession can boast of the same unbroken continuity of methods and of ideals.

CHAUVINISM IN MEDICINE, IN AEQUANIMITAS, 266.

784. *Diseases are not divine or sacred.*

One of the most striking contributions of Hippocrates is the recognition that diseases are only part of the processes of nature, that there is nothing divine or sacred about them.

THE EVOLUTION OF MODERN MEDICINE, 65.

785. The writings of Plato precede Hippocrates.

From the writings of Plato we may gather many details about the status of physicians in his time. It is very evident that the profession was far advanced and had been progressively developing for a long period before Hippocrates, whom we erroneously, yet with a certain propriety, call the *Father of Medicine*.

PHYSIC AND PHYSICIANS AS DEPICTED IN PLATO, IN AEQUANIMITAS, 65.

786. Ancient Israel and Greece cherished rational and esthetic values, but in different proportions.

Modern civilization is the outcome of these two great movements of the mind of man, who to-day is ruled in heart and head by Israel and by Greece.... Not that Israel is all heart, nor Greece all head, for in estimating the human value of the two races, intellect and science are found in Jerusalem and beauty and truth at Athens, but in different proportions.

ISRAEL AND MEDICINE, IN MEN AND BOOKS, 56.

787. The discovery of the circulation of blood was resolved by experiments.

Thousands of men with keen eyes had watched the heart beat, had seen arteries spurt red blood, had seen the black blood flow from the veins, and they had thought and thought and thought of how the heart beat and how the blood flowed, but all in vain until, in a few simple experiments, the problem of its circulation was demonstrated.

THE PATHOLOGICAL INSTITUTE OF A GENERAL HOSPITAL. GLASGOW MED J
1911;76:321-33.

788. Lister's research is true greatness.

Brilliant researches, helpful to our fellows...will come from the University laboratories and the hospitals, but it is difficult to imagine the possibility of another such revolution as that which Joseph Lister [(1827-1912), English surgeon who introduced antisepsis] effected from the wards of the old infirmary—a revolution so far-reaching that we, blessed still by the presence of the Master, while keenly appreciating can scarcely realise its true greatness.

THE PATHOLOGICAL INSTITUTE OF A GENERAL HOSPITAL. GLASGOW MED J
1911;76:321-33.

789. The cause of plagues is infectious.

At the middle of the last century we did not know much more of the actual causes of the great scourges of the race—the plagues, the fever, the pestilences—than did the Greeks. The facts that fevers were catching, that epidemics spread, that infection could remain attached to particles of clothing, etc., all gave support to the view that the actual cause was something alive—a *contagium vivum*.

THE PATHOLOGICAL INSTITUTE OF A GENERAL HOSPITAL. GLASGOW MED J
1911;76:321-33.

790. Advances require revision of understanding.

Even in well-known affections advances are made from time to time that render necessary a revision of our accumulated knowledge, a readjustment of old positions, a removal even of the old landmarks. Perhaps the most remarkable illustration of this is offered by the discovery of the tubercle bacillus. What a *volte face* [about face] for those of us who were teachers before 1881! Happy those who had agility and wit sufficient for the somersault!

THE PRACTICAL VALUES OF LAVERAN'S DISCOVERIES. MED NEWS [PHILADELPHIA]
1895;67:561-4.

8

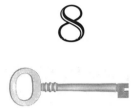

Science and Truth

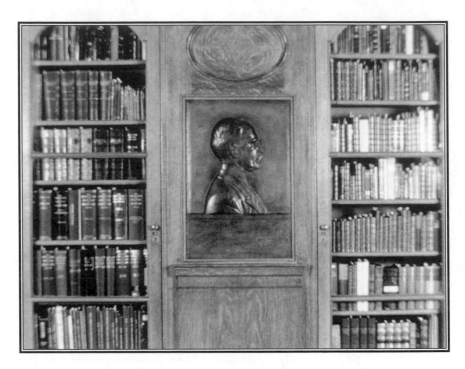

The Osler niche at the Osler Library of the History of Medicine at
McGill University. In the center is a bronze plaque of Osler created by
Frédéric Vernon in Paris in 1905 and known as "the Vernon Plaque."
The ashes of Sir William and Lady Osler are in a casket behind the plaque.
On the left-hand side are Osler's own publications and to the right
is his collection of the works of Sir Thomas Browne, his favorite author.
(Courtesy of the Osler Library of the History of Medicine,
Montreal, Quebec, Canada.)

Science and Truth

Science

791. Balance the rational and the emotional.

To keep his mind sweet, the modern scientific man should be saturated with the Bible and Plato, with Homer, Shakespeare, and Milton; to see life through their eyes may enable him to strike a balance between the rational and the emotional, which is the most serious difficulty of the intellectual life.

SCIENCE AND IMMORTALITY, 42.

792. Science is judged to be a blessing.

And what shall be our final judgment—for or against science? War is more terrible, more devastating, more brutal butchery, and the organisation of the forces of nature has enabled man to wage it on a titanic scale.... To humanity in the gross, she seems a monster, but on the other side is a great credit balance—the enormous number spared the misery of sickness, the unspeakable tortures saved by anaesthesia, the more prompt care of the wounded, the better surgical technique, the lessened time to convalescence, the whole organization of nursing; the wounded soldier would throw his sword into the scale for science—and he is right.

SCIENCE AND WAR. LANCET 1915;2:795-801.

793. Osler's original description of platelets.

Careful investigation of the blood proves that, in addition to the usual elements, there exist pale granular masses, which on closer inspection present a corpuscular appearance. In size they vary greatly from half or quarter that of a white blood-corpuscle, to enormous masses.... They have a compact solid look...while in specimens examined without any reagents the filaments of fibrin adhere to them.

AN ACCOUNT OF CERTAIN ORGANISMS OCCURRING IN THE LIQUOR SANGUINIS. PROC ROY SOC LOND 1874;22:391-8.

794. No progress can compare with the relief of suffering.

Measure as we may the progress of the world—materially, in the advantages of steam electricity, and other mechanical appliances; sociologically, in the great improvement in the conditions of life; intellectually, in the diffusion of education; morally, in a possibly higher standard of ethics—there is no one measure which can compare with the decrease of physical suffering in man, woman, and child when stricken by disease or accident. This is the one fact of supreme personal import to every one of us. This is the Promethean [after Prometheus, Greek titan who stole fire from heaven to give to mankind] gift of the [nineteenth] century to man.

MEDICINE IN THE NINETEENTH CENTURY, IN AEQUANIMITAS, 220.

795. *Medicine has a glorious future.*

And not only in what has been actually accomplished in unravelling the causes of disease, in perfecting methods of prevention, and in wholesale relief of suffering, but also in the unloading of old formulae and in the substitution of the scientific spirit of free inquiry for cast-iron dogmas we see a promise of still greater achievement and of a more glorious future.

CHAUVINISM IN MEDICINE, IN AEQUANIMITAS, 268.

796. *Medicine and science have made major advances.*

To have lived through a revolution, to have seen a new birth of science, a new dispensation of health, reorganized medical schools, remodeled hospitals, a new outlook for humanity, is not given to every generation.

SPECIALISM IN THE GENERAL HOSPITAL. JOHNS HOPKINS HOSP BULL 1913;24:167-71.

797. *The achievements of anesthesia, sanitation, and asepsis cannot be equaled.*

Search the scriptures of human achievement and you cannot find any to equal in beneficence the introduction of Anaesthesia, Sanitation, with all that it includes, and Asepsis—a short half century's contribution towards the practical solution of the problems of human suffering, regarded as eternal and insoluble.

CHAUVINISM IN MEDICINE, IN AEQUANIMITAS, 268.

798. Science leavens the social fabric.

Who runs may read the scroll which reason has placed as a warning over the human menageries: "chained, not tamed." And yet who can doubt that the leaven of science, working in the individual, leavens in some slight degree the whole social fabric. Reason is at least free, or nearly so; the shackles of dogma have been removed, and faith herself, freed from a morganatic alliance [that is, an alliance between the noble and the common], finds in the release great gain.

THE LEAVEN OF SCIENCE, IN AEQUANIMITAS, 94.

799. Experimentation gives control over nature.

The ancients thought as clearly as we do, had greater skills in the arts and in architecture, but they had never learned the use of the great instrument which has given man control over nature—experiment.

THE PATHOLOGICAL INSTITUTE OF A GENERAL HOSPITAL. GLASGOW MED J
1911;76:321-33.

800. Only science and experimentation can reveal the secrets of nature.

Seeing and thinking have done much for human progress; in the sphere of mind and morals everything, and could the world have been saved by armchair philosophy, the Greeks would have done it; but only a *novum organon* [the interpretation of Nature and Man] could do this, the powerful possibilities of which were only revealed when man began to search out the secrets of nature by way of experiment, to use the words of Harvey.

THE PATHOLOGICAL INSTITUTE OF A GENERAL HOSPITAL. GLASGOW MED J
1911;76:321-33.

801. Life is Nature's experiment.

To each of us life is an experiment in Nature's laboratory, and she tests and tries us in a thousand ways, using us and improving us if we serve her turn, ruthlessly dispensing with us if we do not.

THE EVOLUTION OF THE IDEA OF EXPERIMENT IN MEDICINE. TRANSACTIONS OF THE CONGRESS OF AMERICAN PHYSICIANS AND SURGEONS. SEVENTH TRIENNIAL SESSION. NEW HAVEN: BY THE CONGRESS, 1907:7.

802. Experimental medicine and mathematics have solved many problems.

That man can interrogate as well as observe nature was a lesson slowly learned in his evolution. Of the two methods by which he can do this, the mathematical and the experimental, both have been equally fruitful—by the one he has gauged the starry heights and harnessed the cosmic forces to his will; by the other he has solved many of the problems of life and lightened many of the burdens of humanity.

ROLAND C. THE EVOLUTION OF THE IDEA OF EXPERIMENT IN MEDICINE. IN SIR WILLIAM OSLER, 1849-1919: A SELECTION FOR MEDICAL STUDENTS. TORONTO: THE HANNAH INSTITUTE FOR THE HISTORY OF MEDICINE, 1982:103.

803. The beginning of medicine is to wonder.

Like other departments of philosophy, medicine began with an age of wonder. The accidents of disease and the features of death aroused surprise and stimulated interest, and a beginning was made when man first asked in astonishment, Why should these things be?

THE EVOLUTION OF INTERNAL MEDICINE. IN MODERN MEDICINE: ITS THEORY AND PRACTICE. PHILADELPHIA: LEA BROTHERS & CO., 1907:16.

804. The individual may pay the price of breaking with custom.

In departing from any settled opinion or belief, the variation, the change, the break with custom may come gradually; and the way is usually prepared; but the final break is made, as a rule, by some one individual,...who sees with his own eyes, and with an instinct or genius for truth, escapes from the routine in which his fellows live. But he often pays dearly for his boldness.

HARVEY AND HIS DISCOVERY, IN AN ALABAMA STUDENT, 300.

805. To understand science one must trace its development.

To understand clearly our position in any science to-day, we must go back to its beginnings, and trace its gradual development, following certain laws, difficult to interpret and often obscured in the brilliancy of achievements—laws which everywhere illustrate this biography, this human endeavour, working through the long ages; and particularly is this the case with that history of the organized experience of the race which we call science.

HARVEY AND HIS DISCOVERY, IN AN ALABAMA STUDENT, 296.

806. Understand the nature of science.

By scientific I do not mean the acquisition of the bare facts of science, but an understanding of its methods, a realisation of its meaning and an inoculation with its spirit. It is an attitude of mind, a sort of reflex, which at once on the presentation of a problem makes a man burn until its solution is accomplished, until he knows the status of the question among the investigators of the world.

THE RESERVES OF LIFE. ST. MARY'S HOSP GAZ 1907;13:95-8.

807. Science seeks to know and control.

Magic and religion control the uncharted sphere—the supernatural, the superhuman: science seeks to know the world, and through knowing, to control it.

THE EVOLUTION OF MODERN MEDICINE, 5.

808. Progress occurs by clarifying structure and then function.

The determination of structure with a view to the discovery of function has been the foundation of progress.

THE LEAVEN OF SCIENCE, IN AEQUANIMITAS, 85.

809. Science enables one to separate the true from the false.

A devotion to science, a saturation with its spirit, will give you that most precious of all faculties—a sane, cool reason which enables you to sift the true from the false in life and, at the same time, keeps you well in the van of progress.

THE RESERVES OF LIFE. ST. MARY'S HOSP GAZ 1907;13:95-8.

810. Science is accurate observation.

Science has been defined as the habit or faculty of observation…Only a quantitative difference makes observation scientific—accuracy.

THE OLD HUMANITIES AND THE NEW SCIENCE, IN A WAY OF LIFE, 26.

811. An institute is the cerebrum of the infirmary.

An institute is something more than a dead house, and very much more than an ordinary pathological laboratory. It is the cerebrum of the infirmary, the place where the thinking is done, where ideas are nurtured,

where men dream dreams, and thoughts are materialised into researches upon the one great problem that confronts the profession in each
generation—*the nature of disease.*

THE PATHOLOGICAL INSTITUTE OF A GENERAL HOSPITAL. GLASGOW MED J
1911;76:321-33.

812. *Acknowledge our debt to the leaders and workers of science.*

It is well to acknowledge the debt which we every-day practitioners owe
to the great leaders and workers in the scientific branches of our art. We
dwell too much in corners, and, consumed with the petty cares of a
bread-and-butter struggle, forget that outside our routine lie Elysian
fields into which we may never have wandered, the tillage of which is not
done by our hands, but the fruits of which we of the profession and you
of the public fully and freely enjoy.

RUDOLPH VIRCHOW: THE MAN AND THE STUDENT. BOSTON MED SURG J
1891;125:425-7.

813. *The investigator thinks of the future.*

The investigator, to be successful, must start abreast of the knowledge
of the day, and he differs from the teacher, who, living in the present,
expounds only what is current, in that his thoughts must be in the
future, and his ways and work in advance of the day in which he lives.

TEACHER AND STUDENT, IN AEQUANIMITAS, 29-30.

814. *The credit goes to the man who convinces.*

In science the credit goes to the man who convinces the world, not to
the man to whom the idea first occurs.

BEAN WB. SIR WILLIAM OSLER: APHORISMS, 112.

815. Society owes an enormous debt to the pioneers of scientific discovery.

Only a cold-hearted, apathetic, phlegmatic, batrachian [frogs and toads], white-livered generation, with blood congealed in the cold storage of commercialism, could not recognize the enormous debt which we owe to these self-sacrificing miners of science.

SPECIALISM IN THE GENERAL HOSPITAL. JOHNS HOPKINS HOSP BULL 1913;24:167-71.

816. A researcher excels by his merits.

But let the student remember that while influence or party may advance a man in other professions above many superior to himself, the hero in medical research must wholly depend upon his own deservings. To take a foremost place in the wary and critical field of science he must excel.

INTRODUCTORY ADDRESS AT THE OPENING OF THE FORTY-FIFTH SESSION OF THE MEDICAL FACULTY, McGILL COLLEGE. CAN MED SURG J 1877-78;6:193-210.

817. Give credit to others.

Familiarize yourself with the work of others and never fail to give credit to the precursor.

BEAN WB. SIR WILLIAM OSLER: APHORISMS, 71.

818. Others may get credit for the work of someone else.

Too often the reaper is not the sower...Too often the fate of those who labour at some object of the public good is to see their work pass into other hands, and to have others get the credit for enterprises which they have initiated and made possible.

BOOKS AND MEN, IN A WAY OF LIFE, 35.

819. Competition is damaging to scientific work.

Another unpleasant manifestation of collegiate Chauvinism is the outcome, perhaps, of the very keen competition which at present exists in
scientific circles. Instead of a generous appreciation of the work done in
other places, there is a settled hostility and a narrowness of judgment but
little in keeping with the true spirit of science.

CHAUVINISM IN MEDICINE, IN AEQUANIMITAS, 280.

820. Jealousy must be avoided in judging the work of others.

A dark shadow in the scientific life is often thrown by a spirit of jealousy,
and the habit of suspicious, carping criticism. The hall-mark of a small
mind, this spirit should never be allowed to influence our judgment of a
man's work.

VALLERY-RADOT R. THE LIFE OF PASTEUR (INTRODUCTION BY W. OSLER). LONDON:
CONSTABLE AND CO., 1911:9-22.

821. Science will increasingly control the future.

The future belongs to science. More and more she will control the des-
tinies of nations. Already she has them in her crucible and on her bal-
ances. In her new mission to humanity she preaches a new gospel.

VALLERY-RADOT R. THE LIFE OF PASTEUR (INTRODUCTION BY WILLIAM OSLER).
LONDON: CONSTABLE AND CO., 1911:9-22.

822. The acceptance of scientific truth is slow.

To scientific truth alone may the *homo mensura* principle [from
Protagoras, a pre-Socratic philosopher—man is the measure] be applied,
since of all mental treasures of the race it alone compels general acquiescence. That this general acquiescence, this aspect of certainty, is not
reached *per saltum* [through a leap], but is of slow, often of difficult,
growth—marked by failures and frailties, but crowned at last with an

acceptance accorded to no other product of mental activity—is illustrated by every important discovery from Copernicus to Darwin.

HARVEY AND HIS DISCOVERY, IN AN ALABAMA STUDENT, 297.

823. Every scientific truth is met initially by skepticism.

It is one of the great tragedies of life that every truth has to struggle to acceptance against honest but mind-blind students.

THE STUDENT LIFE, IN A WAY OF LIFE, 172.

824. Scientific discovery precedes good medical practice.

The hospital units mint, for current use in the community, the gold wrought by the miners of science.

SPECIALISM IN THE GENERAL HOSPITAL. JOHNS HOPKINS HOSP BULL 1913;24:167-71.

825. A scientific discipline leads to salvation.

To the physician particularly a scientific discipline is an incalculable gift, which leavens his whole life, giving exactness to habits of thought and tempering the mind with that judicious faculty of distrust which can alone, amid the uncertainties of practice, make him wise unto salvation.

THE LEAVEN OF SCIENCE, IN AEQUANIMITAS, 92.

826. Science cannot control emotions.

Science has done much, and will do more, to alleviate the unhappy condition in which so many millions of our fellow-creatures live, and in no way more than in mitigating some of the horrors of disease; but we are too apt to forget that apart from and beyond her domain lie those irresistible forces which alone sway the hearts of men. With reason science never parts company, but with feeling, emotion, passion, what has she to do? They are not of her; they owe her no allegiance. She may study, analyze, and define, she can never control them, and by no possibility can their ways be justified to her.

THE LEAVEN OF SCIENCE, IN AEQUANIMITAS, 93.

827. The patient must benefit from experimental interventions.

We have no right to use patients entrusted to our care for the purpose of experimentation unless direct benefit to the individual is likely to follow. Once this limit is transgressed, the sacred cord which binds physician and patient snaps instantly...enthusiasm for science has, in a few instances, led to regrettable transgression of the rule I have mentioned, but these are mere specks which in no wise blur the brightness of the picture—one of the brightest in the history of human effort—which portrays the incalculable benefits to man from the introduction of experimentation into the art of medicine.

THE EVOLUTION OF THE IDEA OF EXPERIMENT IN MEDICINE. TRANSACTIONS OF THE CONGRESS OF AMERICAN PHYSICIANS AND SURGEONS. SEVENTH TRIENNIAL SESSION. NEW HAVEN: BY THE CONGRESS, 1907:7.

828. In research, concentrate your efforts on a small area.

A little field well-tilled! How much more may come from it than from a large one with its surface only scratched!

WARTHIN AS. OSLER AND THE INTERNATIONAL ASSOCIATION OF MEDICAL MUSEUMS (EDITORIAL). IN ABBOTT ME (ED). SIR WILLIAM OSLER MEMORIAL NUMBER. BULLETIN NO. IX OF THE INTERNATIONAL ASSOCIATION OF MEDICAL MUSEUMS AND JOURNAL OF TECHNICAL METHODS. MONTREAL: PRIVATELY PRINTED, 1926:2.

829. Science has prolonged lives.

Modern science has made to almost everyone of you the present of a few years.

BEAN WB. SIR WILLIAM OSLER: APHORISMS, 111.

830. The practitioner must rely on teachers and investigators.

Science must ever hold with Epicharmus [6th-5th century B.C. Greek comic dramatist] that a judicious distrust and wise scepticism are the sinews of the understanding. And yet the very foundations of belief in almost everything relating to our art rest upon authority. The practitioner cannot always be the judge; the responsibility must often rest with the teachers and investigators, who can only learn in the lessons of history the terrible significance of the word.

BRITISH MEDICINE IN GREATER BRITAIN, IN AEQUANIMITAS, 173.

831. The humanities and the sciences are complementary.

Twin berries on one stem, grievous damage has been done to both in regarding the Humanities and Science in any other light than complemental.

THE OLD HUMANITES AND THE NEW SCIENCE. BRIT MED J 1919;2:1-7.

Truth

832. Truth grows and evolves over time.

Like a living organism, Truth grows, and its gradual evolution may be traced from the tiny germ to the mature product. Never springing, Minerva-like, to full stature at once, Truth may suffer all the hazards incident to generation and gestation. Much of history is a record of the mishaps of truths which have struggled to the birth, only to die or else to wither in premature decay. Or the germ may be dormant for centuries, awaiting the fullness of time.

HARVEY AND HIS DISCOVERY, IN AN ALABAMA STUDENT, 296.

833. *General acceptance of truth takes time.*

The history of the acceptance of any great truth in medicine is an interesting study. A slow, gradual recognition seems essential to permanence and stability.

> On the Study of Tuberculosis. Phila Med J 1900;6:1029-30.

834. *Be satisfied with your best endeavor.*

At the outset do not be worried about this big question—Truth. It is a very simple matter if each one of you starts with the desire to get as much as possible. No human being is constituted to know the truth, the whole truth, and nothing but the truth; and even the best of men must be content with fragments, with partial glimpses, never the full fruition.

> The Student Life, in Aequanimitas, 397-8.

835. *Be satisfied with the best truth available and aware that it may be incomplete.*

The truth is the best you can get with your best endeavour, the best that the best men accept—with this you must learn to be satisfied, retaining at the same time with due humility an earnest desire for an ever larger portion.

> The Student Life, in Aequanimitas, 398.

9

Faith, Religion, Melancholy, Death

- → Faith and Religion

- → Melancholy and Death

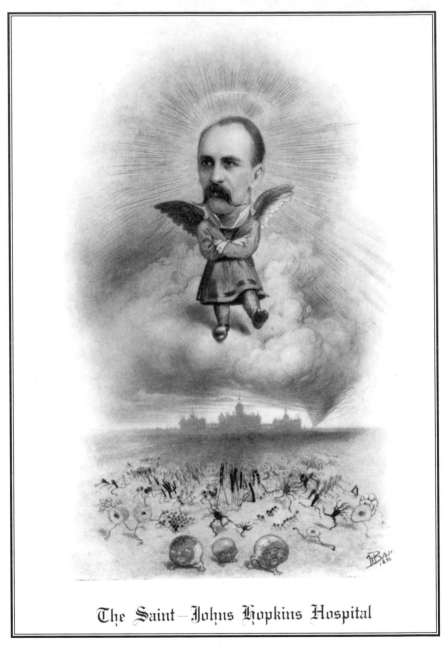

The Saint—Johns Hopkins Hospital

Drawing of William Osler—"The Saint"—Johns Hopkins Hospital by Max Brödel
in 1896. In the foreground, amoebas, malarial parasites, staphylococci, and
streptococci are fleeing but typhoid bacilli are undaunted.
(Courtesy of the Alan Mason Chesney Medical Archives of the Johns Hopkins
Medical Institutions.)

Faith, Religion, Melancholy, Death

Faith and Religion

836. Faith in the doctor can cure.

Faith in the gods or in the saints cures one, faith in little pills another, hypnotic suggestion a third, faith in a plain common doctor a fourth.

MEDICINE IN THE NINETEENTH CENTURY, IN AEQUANIMITAS, 259.

837. Faith in the physician can work miracles.

As a profession, consciously or unconsciously, more often the latter, *faith* has been one of our most valuable assets, and Galen expressed a great truth when he said, "He cures most successfully in whom the people have the greatest confidence." It is in these cases of neurasthenia and psychasthenia, the weak brothers and the weak sisters, that the personal character of the physician comes into play, and once let him gain the confidence of the patient, he can work just the same sort of miracles as Our Lady of Lourdes [French shrine of healing] or Ste. Anne de Beaupré [Quebec shrine of faith healing].

THE PRINCIPLES AND PRACTICE OF MEDICINE, 1095.

838. Faith underlies the healing in many settings.

While we doctors often overlook or are ignorant of our own faith-cures, we are just a wee bit too sensitive about those performed outside our ranks. We have never had, and cannot expect to have a monopoly in this panacea, which is open to all, free as the sun, and which may make of every one in certain cases, as was the Lacedemonian [a person from Sparta, a Greek city in the Peloponnesus] of Homer's day, "a good physician out of Nature's grace."

MEDICINE IN THE NINETEENTH CENTURY, IN AEQUANIMITAS, 259.

839. The power of faith.

Nothing in life is more wonderful than faith—the one great moving force which we can neither weigh in the balance nor test in the crucible. Intangible as the ether, ineluctable as gravitation, the radium of the moral and mental spheres, mysterious, indefinable, known only by its effects, faith pours out an unfailing stream of energy while abating nor jot nor tittle of its potency.

THE FAITH THAT HEALS. BRIT MED J 1910;1:1470-2.

840. A man must have faith in himself.

A man must have faith in himself to be of any use in the world. There may be very little on which to base it—no matter, but faith in one's powers, in one's mission is essential to success. Confidence once won, the rest follows naturally; and with a strong faith in himself a man becomes a local centre for its radiation.

THE FAITH THAT HEALS. BRIT MED J 1910;1:1470-2.

841. Faith is the great stock in trade in the practice of medicine.

A third noteworthy feature in modern treatment has been a return to psychical methods of cure, in which faith in something is suggested to the patient. After all, faith is the great lever of life. Without it, man can do nothing; with it, even with a fragment, as a grain of mustard seed, all things are possible to him. Faith in us, faith in our drugs and methods, is the great stock in trade of the profession.

MEDICINE IN THE NINETEENTH CENTURY, IN AEQUANIMITAS, 258-9.

842. Acknowledge the value of a belief in a hereafter.

Though his philosophy finds nothing to support it...the scientific student should be ready to acknowledge the value of a belief in a hereafter as an asset to human life. In the presence of so many mysteries which have been unveiled, in the presence of so many yet unsolved, he cannot be dogmatic and deny the possibility of a future state.... He will recognize that amid the ebb and flow of human misery, a belief in the resurrection of the dead and the life of the world to come is the rock of safety to which many of the noblest of his fellows have clung.

SCIENCE AND IMMORTALITY, 39-40.

843. Faith is a precious commodity.

In all ages the prayer of faith has healed the sick.... We enjoy, I say, no monopoly in the faith business. The faith with which we work, the faith, indeed, which is available to-day in everyday life, has its limitations. It will not raise the dead; it will not put in a new eye in place of a bad one,...nor will it cure cancer or pneumonia, or knit a bone; but...such as we find it, faith is a most precious commodity, without which we should be very badly off.

MEDICINE IN THE NINETEENTH CENTURY, IN AEQUANIMITAS, 259-60.

844. An inexhaustible supply of faith remains.

The most active manifestations [of faith] are in the countless affiliations which man in his evolution has worked out with the unseen, with the invisible powers, whether of light or of darkness, to which from time immemorial he has erected altars and shrines.... Creeds pass; an inexhaustible supply of faith remains.

THE FAITH THAT HEALS. BRIT MED J 1910;1:1470-2.

845. Mental healing can be valuable.

While in general use for centuries, one good result of the recent development of mental healing has been to call attention to its great value as a measure to be carefully and scientifically applied in suitable cases. My experience has been that of the unconscious rather than the deliberate faith healer. Phenomenal, even what could be called miraculous, cures are not very uncommon. Like others, I have had cases any one of which, under suitable conditions, could have been worthy of a shrine or made the germ of pilgrimage.

THE FAITH THAT HEALS. BRIT MED J 1910;1:1470-2.

846. The influence of faith is not apparent to the senses.

When reason calls in vain and arguments fall on deaf ears, the still small voice of a life lived in the full faith of another may charm like the lute of Orpheus [Greek poet-musician with magical powers] and compel an unwilling assent by a strong, indefinable attraction, not to be explained in words, outside the laws of philosophy—a something which is not apparent to the senses, and which is manifest only in its effects.

SCIENCE AND IMMORTALITY, 37.

847. *Science cannot supply the heart.*

The man of science is in a sad quandary to-day. He cannot but feel that the emotional side to which faith leans makes for all that is bright and joyous in life. Fed on the dry husks of facts, the human heart has a hidden want which science cannot supply; as a steady diet it is too strong and meaty, and hinders rather than promotes harmonious mental metabolism.

SCIENCE AND IMMORTALITY, 41.

848. *Mixing science and faith can be treacherous.*

One and all of you will have to face the ordeal of every student in this generation who sooner or later tries to mix the waters of science with the oil of faith. You can have a great deal of both if you only keep them separate. The worry comes from the attempt at mixture.

THE MASTER-WORD IN MEDICINE, IN AEQUANIMITAS, 365.

849. *Science cannot explain things unseen.*

Science is organized knowledge, and knowledge is of things we see. Now the things that are seen are temporal; of the things that are unseen science knows nothing, and has at present no means of knowing anything.

SCIENCE AND IMMORTALITY, 40-1.

850. *Faith is important to believers in immortality.*

On the question of immortality the only enduring enlightenment is through faith.

SCIENCE AND IMMORTALITY, 39.

851. *As we grow old, many of us have less belief in a future life.*

And the eventide of life is not always hopeful; on the contrary, the older we grow, the less fixed, very often, is the belief in a future life.

SCIENCE AND IMMORTALITY, 13.

852. *Belief in immortality varies.*

While accepting a belief in immortality and accepting the phases and forms of the prevailing religion, an immense majority live practically uninfluenced by it, except in so far as it ministers to a wholesale dissonance between the inner and the outer life, and diffuses an atmosphere of general insincerity. A second group, larger, perhaps, to-day than ever before in history, put the supernatural altogether out of man's life, and regard the hereafter as only one of the many inventions he has sought out for himself. A third group, ever small and select, lay hold with the anchor of faith upon eternal life as the controlling influence in this one.

SCIENCE AND IMMORTALITY, 8.

853. *Spirits and demons may bring comfort or sorrow.*

It may be questioned whether more comfort or sorrow has come to the race since man peopled the unseen world with spirits to bless and demons to damn him.

SCIENCE AND IMMORTALITY, 27-8.

854. *Osler's confession of faith.*

Some of you will wander through all phases [of religious conviction], to come at last, I trust, to the opinion of Cicero [1st century B.C. Roman statesman and philosopher], who had rather be mistaken with Plato than be in the right with those who deny altogether the life after death; and this is my own *confessio fidei.*

SCIENCE AND IMMORTALITY, 43.

855. Clergymen support nostrums and humbuggery.

I suppose as a body, clergymen are better educated than any other, yet they are notorious supporters of all the nostrums and humbuggery with which the daily and religious papers abound.

TEACHING AND THINKING, IN AEQUANIMITAS, 124.

856. Clergy should not try to deal with the hysterical.

The less the clergy have to do with the bodily complaints of neurasthenic and hysterical persons the better for their peace of mind and the reputation of the cloth.

THE TREATMENT OF DISEASE. CAN LANCET 1909;42:899-912.

857. Christian Science is misleading.

Never before in a history surcharged with examples of credulity has so monstrously puerile a belief [Christian Science] been exploited. To deny the existence of disease, to deny the reality of pain, to disregard all physical measures of relief, to sweep away in a spiritual ecstasy the accumulated wisdom of centuries in a return to Oriental mysticism—these, indeed, expressed a revolt from the materialism of the latter half of the nineteenth century at once weird, perhaps not unexpected, and, to a student of human nature, just a bit comic.

THE FAITH THAT HEALS. BRIT MED J 1910;2:1470-2.

858. Begin the day with Christ and prayer.

Begin the day with Christ and His prayer—you need no other. Creedless, with it you have religion; creed-stuffed, it will leaven any theological dough in which you stick. As the soul is dyed by the thoughts, let no day pass without contact with the best literature of the world.

A WAY OF LIFE, IN A WAY OF LIFE, 248.

Melancholy and Death

859. Sorrow is inevitable.

Sorrows and griefs are companions sure sooner or later to join us on our pilgrimage, and we have become perhaps more sensitive to them, and perhaps less amenable to the old time remedies of the physicians of the soul; but the pains and woes of the body, to which we doctors minister, are decreasing at an extraordinary rate, and in a way that makes one fairly gasp in hopeful anticipation.

TEACHING AND THINKING, IN AEQUANIMITAS, 118.

860. Melancholy is a loss of life's sweetness.

Melancholy may be defined as a state of mind in which a man is so out of touch with his environment that life has lost its sweetness.

ROBERT BURTON: THE MAN, HIS BOOKS, HIS LIBRARY, IN A WAY OF LIFE, 65.

861. The unhappy choose death.

The worries and stress of business, the pangs of misprized love, the anguish of religious despair, make an increasing number of unhappy ones choose death rather than a bitter life.

ROBERT BURTON: THE MAN, HIS BOOKS, HIS LIBRARY, IN A WAY OF LIFE, 86.

862. The best antidote to melancholy is unselfish devotion to others.

Let us bury the worries of yesterday in the work of to-day. Some little tincture of Saturn may be allowed in our hearts, but never in our faces. Sorrow and sadness must come to each one—it is our lot;…We can best oppose any tendency to melancholy by an active life of unselfish devotion to others.

ROBERT BURTON: THE MAN, HIS BOOKS, HIS LIBRARY, IN A WAY OF LIFE, 87-8.

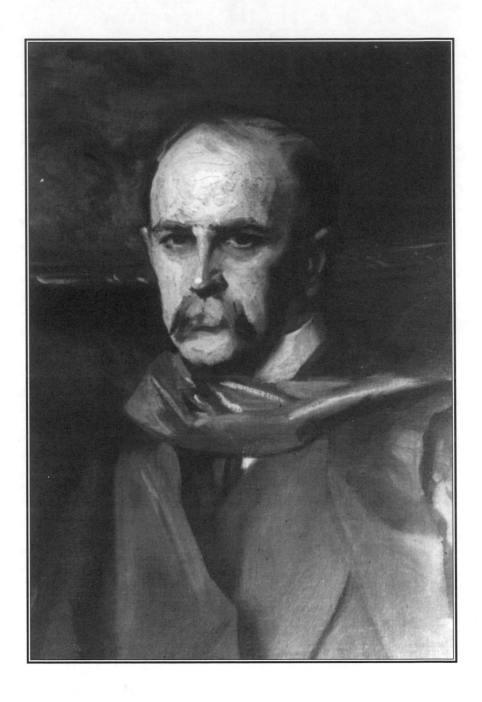

Sir William Osler, detail from *The Four Doctors* by John Singer Sargent,
oil on canvas, 1907. (Courtesy of the Alan Mason Chesney Medical Archives
of the Johns Hopkins Medical Institutions; photo by Aaron Levin.)

An Osler Chronology

COMPILED BY

MARK E. SILVERMAN, MD

Sir William Osler is often considered to be the most admired and influential physician of the 20th century and the father of American medicine. Even 90 years after his death, his name is still remembered, he is widely quoted, and he is considered to be the ideal role model.

1849   Born July 12 in Bond Head, Ontario, Canada, near Toronto, the eighth of nine children of Featherstone and Ellen Osler. His father was an Anglican minister. The family was originally from Cornwall, England.

1857   Family moves to Dundas, Ontario.

1866   Kicked out of grammar school for locking geese in room, covering the chimney. At the age 16, needing discipline for his pranks, the mischievous William is sent to a private boarding school at Weston, Ontario. There he is influenced by the headmaster, Father WA Johnson, an ardent natural scientist, and James Bovell, a leading physician and enthusiastic microscopist. Osler develops a keen interest in biology.

1867   Osler attends Trinity College, Toronto, initially planning to become a minister. He lives with James Bovell, attends his medical rounds, reads from his extensive library, and instead enters Toronto Medical School in 1868.

1870   Osler tranfers to McGill Univ., a four year medical school with better clinical facilities. There he meets Dr. Palmer Howard, the third of his important mentors, who stimulates his interest in reading and pathology.

1872   Graduates McGill with MD degree.

1872-74   Osler travels to England where he works under Dr. Burdon Sanderson and publishes an original description of platelets. After England, he attends clinics in Berlin and Vienna, studying under Rudolph Virchow, Traube, Rokitansky and other great German clinician-teacher-investigators. He is exposed to "Innere Medzin" (Internal Medicine), a concept based on recent advances in pathophysiology, chemistry, and bacteriology which Osler later introduces in the U.S.

1874-75   Age 25, Osler is appointed Lecturer, then in 1875 Professor of Clinical Medicine at McGill. "The baby professor." Teaches physiology and pathology, performs 1000 autopsies, starts a physiology lab, supervises a smallpox ward, becomes a popular teacher and education reformer.

1884   Age 35, Osler flips a coin and succeeds Dr. William Pepper as Chief of Medicine, University of Pennsylvania. Meets Grace Revere Gross, great granddaughter of Paul Revere, wife of surgeon Samuel Gross. Osler's reputation grows as a teacher and clinician.

1887   John Shaw Billings offers him the Chief of Medicine position at the planned new medical school at Johns Hopkins. "Will you take charge of the medical department at JHH? See Welch about the details. We are to open very soon. I am busy today. Good morning." This would be his great opportunity to establish a clinic on the Germanic model. His valedictory address at Penn in 1889 is titled "Aequanimitas." Eli Lilly would distribute 150,000 copies (1932-1953).

1889   Age 40, Osler is the new Chief of Medicine at Johns Hopkins along with Welch, Kelly, and Halstead. "A model of its kind," a university with its own hospital, 4-year medical school, able to produce men to do original research.

1889-92   Medical school not open for 4 years. Osler lives in the hospital and writes *Principles and Practice of Medicine*, published in 1892, which will go through 16 editions and sell 500,000 copies over 55 years. Marvel of clarity, profound influence. Rockefeller story. Marries, at age 42, the widow Grace Revere Gross: "Here's the book, now will you take the man?" Story of registering as EY Davis, deaf visitor.

1889-1905   At JHH, Osler develops the first housestaff system, introduces students to bedside teaching, writes many of his 1600 articles and essays, becomes a celebrated physician with a large consultant practice. He is a dedicated bibliophile whose collection, later given to McGill, will number 7600 books. Bibliotecha Osleriana. Son Revere born 1895.

1904   Osler, burdened by practice and demands, is burned out. Offered Regius Chair of Medicine at Oxford University, England. "Better to go in a steamer than in a pinebox."

1905   Age 56, Osler delivers controversial farewell address, "L'Envoi." Mentioning "The Fixed Period" by Troloppe. "Chloroform at 60!" To Oslerize means to put a man to death (Mencken). Oslers move to Oxford to live at 13 Norham Gardens, "The Open Arms." Dinners three times a week, up to 80 guests. Osler organizes clinic at Radcliffe Infirmary, becomes President of the Classical Association and the British Hospital Association, and is active in many other British organizations.

1911   Osler is conferred a baronetcy by King George V and becomes Sir William Osler.

1914   Osler is appointed Consultant to British Army. World War I begins. Rounds at Colchester.

1917   Osler is devastated when his son Revere is killed at Flanders Field, Belgium, literally dying in the hands of Harvey Cushing. "The Fates do not allow the good fortune that has followed me to go to the grave. Call no man happy till he dies."

"In Flanders fields the poppies blow / Between the crosses, row on row / That mark our place; and in the sky / The larks, still bravely singing, fly / Scarce heard amidst the guns below.

We are the Dead. Short days ago / We lived, felt dawn, saw sunset glow, / Loved, and were loved, and now we lie / In Flanders Fields.

Take up our quarrel with the foe: / To you from failing hands we throw / the Torch; be yours to hold it high. / If ye break faith with us who die / We shall not sleep, though poppies grow / In Flanders Fields."

JOHN MCRAE (1872-1918),
CANADIAN PHYSICIAN AND ONE OF OSLER'S HOUSESTAFF.

1919   Age 70, December 29, Sir William Osler dies of pneumonia and empyema.

It has been said that Oslerian-style medicine is no longer possible under the urgencies and restrictions of managed care. Although there is some truth to this, I believe that this is a defeatist attitude and that the privileges and satisfactions of being a physician are eternal, endlessly rewarding, as germane today as they were then, and that we can still strive to be William Osler at the bedside.

"I have had three personal ideals. One to do the day's work well and not to bother about tomorrow. It has been urged that this is not a satisfactory ideal.... To it, more than to anything else, I owe whatever success I have had—to this power of settling down to the day's work and trying to do it well to the best of one's ability, and letting the future take care of itself. The second ideal has been to act the Golden Rule, as far as in me lay, towards my professional brethren and towards the patients committed to my care. And the third has been to cultivate such a measure of equanimity as would enable me to bear success with humility, the affection of my friends without pride and to be ready when the day of sorrow and grief came to meet it with the courage befitting a man."

William Osler
"L'Envoi" in Aequanimitas

"When he came to die, Osler was, in a very real sense, the greatest physician of our time. He was one of Nature's chosen. Good looks, distinction, blithe manners, a sunbright personality, radiant with kind feeling and good will towards his fellow men, an Apollonian poise, swiftness and surety of thought and speech. Every gift of the gods was his; and to these were added careful training, unsurpassed clinical ability, the widest knowledge of his subject, the deepest interest in everything human, and a serene hold on his fellows that was as a seal set upon them. His enthusiasm for his calling was boundless."

Fielding Garrison

"Sir William Osler is the most famous and influential physician of the early twentieth century. His life can be seen in brief as the fulfillment of two dreams. As a young man he determined to become a great teacher of clinical medicine. His 1892 textbook, *The Principles and Practice of Medicine*, set a new standard and greatly advanced scientific medicine. Having realized his first dream by his early forties, he then set out, perhaps subconsciously at first, to reconcile the emerging new medical science with the old humanities. His unique blend of clinical competence, easy familiarity with the liberal arts, energy, charisma, and idealism made him something of a symbol of humanism in medicine for physicians and laypersons alike."

Charles S. Bryan
Osler: Inspirations from a Great Physician
New York: Oxford University Press, 1997

"Much more than a physician, Osler was a literate, inspiring, humanist in science. His essays and addresses about the medical life, past, present, and future, were widely read and appreciated for their blending of scientific and literary knowledge with high idealism and sensible advice about getting on with the daily grind. In both his writings and his personal life, and through a prism of tragedy in the Great War, Osler seemed to embody the art of living."

Michael Bliss
William Osler: A Life in Medicine
New York: Oxford University Press, 1999

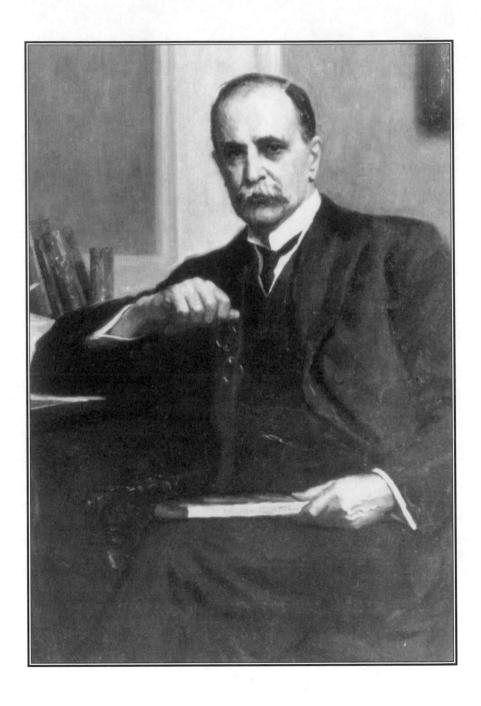

Photograph of the *Portrait of Sir William Osler*
by Seymour Thomas, painted in 1908.
(Courtesy of Earl Nation.)

Frequently Cited Sources

BEAN WB. Sir William Osler: Aphorisms from His Bedside Teachings and Writings. Springfield, IL: Charles C Thomas; 1968.

CAMAC CNB. Counsels and Ideals, from the Writings of William Osler, 2nd ed. Boston: Houghton Mifflin; 1929.

CUSHING H. The Life of Sir William Osler. London: Oxford University Press; 1940 [1-vol reprint of 2-vol first edition (1925)].

OSLER W. Aequanimitas, With Other Addresses to Medical Students, Nurses and Practitioners of Medicine, 3rd ed. Philadelphia: P Blakiston; 1932.

OSLER W. An Alabama Student and Other Biographical Essays. London: Henry Frowde; 1908.

OSLER W. The Evolution of Modern Medicine. New Haven: Yale University Press; 1921.

OSLER W. Introductory Lecture on the Opening of the Forty-Fifth Session of the Medical Faculty, McGuill University. Montreal: Dawson Brothers; 1877.

OSLER W. Lectures on Angina Pectoris and Allied States. New York: D Appleton; 1901.

OSLER W. Men and Books. Durham, NC: Sacrum Press; 1987.

OSLER W. The Principles and Practice of Medicine, 7th ed. New York: D Appleton; 1909.

OSLER W. Science and Immortality. Boston: Houghton Mifflin; 1905.

OSLER W. A Way of Life and Selected Writings of Sir William Osler. New York: Dover Publications; 1951.

THAYER WS. Osler and Other Papers. Baltimore: Johns Hopkins University Press; 1931.

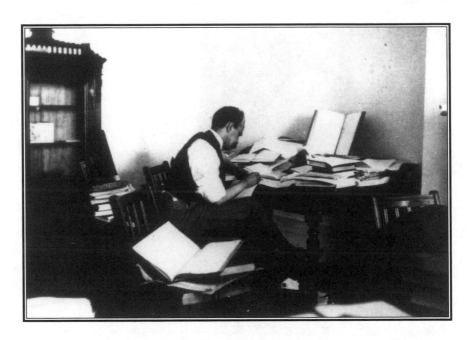

William Osler in 1891 working on
The Principles and Practice of Medicine
at Johns Hopkins Hospital.
(Courtesy of the Osler Library of the History of Medicine,
Montreal, Quebec, Canada)

Index

N.B. Entries refer to quotation number.

K

Keratoses, seborrheic, 451
Kidney, capillaries of, 411
Kindness, 132, 160, 164
Kipling, Rudyard, 5, 90, 258
Knowledge
    absorption of, 104
    of basic science, 179
    contributions to, 181
    of disease, 340, 349
    enlargement of boundaries of, 693
    full, 610
    lack of, 251
    medical students' acquisition of, 575
    men's possession of, 632
    mind's acquisition of, 634
    organized, 849
    of pathology, 338
    practical, 605
    pretension to, 15
    real, 605
    relationship to experience, 330
    relationship to love, 604
    revision of, 790
    specialization-related expansion of, 264
    students' quest for, 573
    as subject of training, 632
    superficial, 314
    teachers' creation of, 725
    teachers' possession of, 696, 699
    as wisdom, 606, 609

L

Labeling, 262, 351
Labor, 194
Laboratories
    experimental, 602
    pathological, 811
Ladies, 150
Language, of healing, 178
Laparotomy, 477
Laughter, 28, 29
Law enforcement, 627
Law (profession), 345
Laws, 805
    of cellular life, 339
    of change, 678
    of health, 170
    of nature, 362
    universal, 326
    of universities, 579
Lawyers, 205
Laziness, 21. See also Idleness
    intellectual, 13, 273
Lead poisoning, 299
Leaders, 60, 812
Learning, 3, 188
    at the bedside, 611, 624
    from errors and mistakes, 618, 620
    lifelong, 641
    from patients, 616, 618
    from teachers, 593
        examinations as hindrance to, 686
        excessive, 572
        lifelong, 560
        through observation, 294
Leaven, 194, 204
Lechery, 470

Lectures, 597, 598, 706, 708, 709, 716, 718, 726
Legislation, 468
Legs, examination of, 304
Leiodermic, 23
Lessons, 615, 616
Leukemia, 487
Leukocytosis, 440
Libraries, 240, 645, 646, 657
Life. *See also* Existence
    battlefield of, 594
    brightening of, 28
    calm, 59
    day-tight compartments in, 123, 124
    direction in, 565
    engines of, 258
    enjoyment of, 61
    facts of, 342
    fire of, 190
    as a habit, 56
    happy, 60
    higher, 85
    institutional, 195
    intellectual, 791
    irritations in, 23
    "middleman" of, 411
    mission of, 276
    modern, as arteriosclerosis cause, 365
    "music" of, 29
    as nature's experiment, 801
    observation of, 315
    one-day-at-a-time approach to, 124
    pace of, 365
    perfect, 57
    philosophy of, 41, 585
    practical, 52
    probability as rule of, 488
    professional, 230
    quiet, 57, 123
    relationship to work, 106
    routine in, 117
    secret of, 105
    simple, 186
    slower approach to, 258
    "struck sharp on Death," 369
    of the student, 582
    talisman of, 106
    of teachers, 722
    temperate, 186
    tragedies of, 359
    trials of, 42
    upright, 589
    useful, 176
    variability in, 324
    vascular "rivers" of, 366
    views of, 55
    in the wards, 672
    work of, 625
Lifespan, 363. *See also* Longevity
Lifestyle, 258, 263, 496–506
    as arteriosclerosis cause, 361, 365
    diet, 496–506
    exercise, 507–509
    for longevity, 506
    vices, 510–523
Listening
    to heart murmurs, 307
    to patients, 287
Lister, Joseph, 758, 788
Literature, 782. *See also* Books
    as source of ideas, 678
    as source of knowledge, 610
Littleness, 604

About the Editors

MARK E. SILVERMAN, MD, is Professor Emeritus at Emory University and Chief of Cardiology at the Fuqua Heart Center, Piedmont Hospital, Atlanta. He is Past-President of the American Osler Society and co-editor of *British Cardiology in the Twentieth Century*. His major interests lie in practicing and teaching the art of bedside cardiology and the history of medicine.

T. JOCK MURRAY, MD, is Professor Emeritus, Dalhousie University, Halifax, Nova Scotia and former Dean of Medicine and founder of the Medical Humanities Program at Dalhousie. He is Past-President of the American Osler Society, the author of *Multiple Sclerosis: the History of a Disease*, and the co-author of *Medicine in Quotations: Views of Health and Disease Through the Ages*.

CHARLES S. BRYAN, MD, is the Heyward Gibbes Distinguished Professor of Internal Medicine at The University of South Carolina School of Medicine. He is Secretary-Treasurer of the American Osler Society, and the author of *Osler: Inspirations from a Great Physician*.